PSYCHED
TO BE
SKINNY

PSYCHED
TO BE
SKINNY

How to Stop Emotional Eating, Enjoy Healthy Weight Loss & Keep It Off for Life!

Dr. Denise Wood, MA, PsyD & Susie Garcia, RDN

SAME PAGE PUBLISHING

Published 2014
Printed in the United States of America
ISBN: 978-1-939825-00-1
Library of Congress Control Number: 2013920486

Contents

Preface

DENISE: We have all been there—depressed, anxiety-ridden, haunted by ghosts of the past and present. These feelings can bring out the Depressed Eater, the Anxious Eater, the Situational Eater, the Bored Eater, the Recently Dumped Eater, the Fat is My Shelter Eater, the Period Eater, the Peer Pressure Eater, and the I Deserve It Eater. All of us have been one of these eaters at some time in our lives.

After having obtained a master's degree in psychology and a doctorate in clinical psychology, I can say that I have finally learned to master my mind and body—and to help my clients do the same. I have established a comfort level with myself; I feel at ease being me. I'm in my forties, have two kids, and have been married for fifteen-plus years. I own my own corporation, Dr. Denise Wood, LLC, and I was in a recent issue of *Supermodels Unlimited Magazine*. I was also the second runner-up for Mrs. Minnesota 2008, and was a sought-out finalist for the longest-running reality show in the United States in April 2011.

I taught aerobics for Bally's U.S. Swim & Fitness for

twenty years. Now I spend my time racing Porsches, slalom skiing, hiking, biking, rock climbing, scuba diving, reading and—most importantly—spending time with family and friends. Thank you for taking this journey with us!

Susie: Like Denise, maintaining a healthy lifestyle, body, and mind is important to me. Many of my clients come to me seeking nutritional counseling in order to lose weight, manage their diabetes, or lower their cholesterol—but what I often find is that multiple behavioral issues are involved in the nutrition choices they make, and that in order to motivate them to make manageable changes in their diet and lifestyle, we have to address those behaviors.

I own and operate a private practice in the San Francisco Bay Area, Nutrition For Your Lifestyle, and have more than twenty years of experience as a dietitian. I work with individuals, families, and businesses, which has provided me valuable insight into the nutritional needs of a variety of people. I've also had the fabulous opportunity of teaching new chefs nutrition and food safety at the Culinary Institute of America in St. Helena, California, and I was recently selected as the official Dietitian/Nutritionist for the San Francisco Bulls hockey team.

Opening my practice in California was a "starting over" step for me—one that I took after finally leaving an abusive marriage. Even when my marriage was at its worst, however, I was always able to maintain my weight and health and to feel good about myself. I have not won any beauty pageants like Denise, but I do consistently hear that I don't look my age—something that is always a pleasure to hear! I am happily remarried now, and I enjoy running, yoga, Pilates, reading, cooking, and taking quick trips to wine country (Napa is only a thirty-minute drive away!) to enjoy fabulous local and sustainable dining, wines, and the company of friends.

DENISE: Susie and I feel that between the two of us we have figured out how to show people how to become the total package. Our approach is about combining mind and body work with cognitive behavioral exercises. We are not about dieting—we are about stable mental health and stable eating. Both of us have stayed at about the same weight throughout our lives; we are not yo-yo dieters, and we are not the magic pill that you can use to lose weight you will quickly gain back. We are weight stabilizers, and we want to teach you to be that as well. We believe that learning weight control from individuals who know how to effectively deal with mental health through stable food and mental health properties is far more effective than learning to shed pounds quickly from individuals who fluctuate in their weight (like many celebrities we all know!).

Regardless of your age or gender, you, too, can have it all. It's all about whole body and mind wellness. Let us help you to love who you are, and you will become a dynamic force for all who come into contact with you. In order to obtain this goal, however, you have to commit to sticking with our program completely— mind, body, and soul. We have a vision for you, but you have to participate fully in order to realize it. You can be physically strong; you can be at the top of your game mentally. You need to believe in yourself, whether you are extroverted or introverted, anxious or laid back, or something in between. Believe in you and your right to be yourself. Once this is established, you will be ready to undergo a mind, body, and soul transformation that will be equaled by none.

Introduction:
How to Use This Book

As you go through this journey with us, we know you will see amazing results. As we walk you along the path of the successful, however, please keep in mind that you are an individual and that you know better than anyone else what is right for you. You may identify most strongly with one of the eating types in this book. But the truth is, we have all been more than one of these types of eaters at some time or another in our lives. You could be a Bored Eater one day but a Depressed or Anxious Eater the next—or you could be two types of eaters simultaneously (if, for instance, you're a Recently Dumped Eater and you're trying to get your significant other back but they won't return your voicemails, text messages, e-mails, Facebook comments, tweets, Snapchats, or smoke signals, and that's making you an Anxious Eater, too!).

With this in mind, feel free to visit as many chapters as are relevant for you. We are merely giving you examples of what may work for you at several different periods in your life. If you need to venture backward or forward as you read this book, please feel free to do so. Don't feel you have to choose one type for yourself and stick to it. Note as well that this book is *not* a weight loss book — rather, it is a book on how to look and feel your best, both physically and emotionally. We don't want you to go on some yo-yo diet where your weight fluctuates up and down, and we don't want you to starve yourself. What we do want is for you to have a stable weight that you are pleased with, which is why we are giving you healthy alternatives to the foods you may currently be eating.

Not everyone who struggles with unhealthy eating habits fits into one category. Therefore, no one diet will work for everyone. We are firm believers in the idea that everyone eats for different reasons — and that figuring out what those reasons are is the first step toward being healthy without going hungry. Know that this ain't your momma's diet book, and that you won't be eating only cabbage soup or grapefruit by the time we're done with you. What you will be doing, though, is changing your eating habits for the better in a sustainable, and even enjoyable, way.

The solution-focused and cognitive behavioral exercises you'll find on the following pages are meant to be used as weapons against your unhealthy eating habits. They will help you steer clear of unhealthy foods, and they will help you stop yourself from overeating. They will help you visualize your healthy self, and they will help you develop a more positive attitude about food in general. Feel free to modify any of these exercises to better suit your needs. Remember, what's most important is that you find the therapeutic tools here that work for *you*.

Have a fabulous time being happier, healthier, and more physically fit. We have faith in you. You are mentally and physically stronger than you think. You can do it. Now let's get started!

1

The Depressed Eater

The Depressed Eater is the eater that eats due to feelings of hopelessness and helplessness. The Depressed Eater feels a need to fill an emotional void, and their primary way of coping with depression is with food. The Depressed Eater may have been taken to Dairy Queen or McDonald's as a child or adolescent when their team lost or when they were feeling down in the dumps; maybe the Depressed Eater went straight for the chips and Twinkies when they came home from a hard day at school. In whatever way, food was probably used to address any discomforts that the Depressed Eater might have endured in their younger years.

As Depressed Eaters grow older, they continue to self-medicate with their food of choice, and inevitably begin to gain weight. The weight gain makes them more depressed which leads to more bouts of eating. The Depressed Eater often feels guilty after they have indulged in food that is unhealthy, and tends to fall even more deeply into depression when confronted with their lack of control over their emotions and food intake. They are very hard on themselves and feel like failures when they eat things they know they should not have eaten. (If you are part of a Depressed Eater's life, you should be cautious about what you say to them about their eating habits.)

Some Depressed Eaters have lost someone or something dear to them—a parent, a significant other, a child, a job—that has triggered their negative behavior patterns. Other Depressed Eaters suffer from chemical imbalances in the brain—a lack of serotonin or norepinephrine. When a Depressed Eater is dealing with both a chemical imbalance in the brain *and* a social stressor, it's even more difficult for them to manage their emotional state.

The Depressed Eater will often use their weight as an excuse not to go to social or business engagements, saying that they are too heavy and do not feel comfortable in their bodies. This self-imposed isolation prompts them to become more depressed, which leads to further isolation—which in turn leads to more feelings of hopelessness and helplessness.

The best antidote for the Depressed Eater is to try to stay active to keep serotonin levels up. Depression is not something to take lightly. If you are feeling suicidal or homicidal, or are in danger of injuring yourself, please contact your mental health provider immediately—and if you do not have one, call 911 and inform them about your situation.

If you're a Depressed Eater, you need to:

- Seek education from a mental health professional so you can find out what is causing you to be a Depressed Eater. You may also want to look into going on an antidepressant.

- Identify your predisposition for/history of eating as an emotional response.

- Think about how you have coped with difficult situations without turning to unhealthy eating habits in the past.

- Identify factors that exacerbate your depressed eating.

- Educate yourself on good nutrition.

- Get regular physical exercise to release tension and decrease your desire to eat.

- Journal your feelings so you can vent about and clarify your problems, and to facilitate your problem-solving skills.

- Reduce the food stimuli in your house to decrease cravings by removing your favorite unhealthy foods.

- Avoid driving or walking by your favorite eating establishments.

- Always give yourself positive feedback when you successfully avoid depressed eating . . . you deserve it!

Cognitive Behavioral Exercises for the Depressed Eater

When feeling the need to eat following a depressed episode, do something active: go for a walk or call a supportive friend, for example. Read a book about proper nutrition habits and try to establish them for yourself. The Depressed Eater should avoid triggers that make them want to eat foods that are unhealthy. You may want to take a different route home, for instance, if it will help you avoid your favorite fattening foods. Do something out of character such as trying rock climbing or going to a comedy club to help yourself forget about your desire to eat unhealthy foods. Join a group therapy session on depressed eating.

Solution-Focused Exercises for the Depressed Eater

If you could wave a magic wand and create the mind and body that you wish you had, what you would feel and look like? Imagine what it would be like to be a mentally and physically healthy person.

Physical Exercise for the Depressed Eater

If you are depressed, you will want to see a medical doctor to identify any medical issues you might have before focusing on getting into good physical shape. Hypothyroidism, for example—something that physical exercise can't help with—can sometimes be at the root of a person becoming depressed and gaining weight.

When you do begin exercising, you'll want to start

out slow and not make your goals too high as failure can increase depression and cause even more depressed eating. If you have not exercised in a while, start by simply going for a walk around the block. If you are in fairly good shape, try going for a jog with a trusted friend or relative. Get on a treadmill or elliptical machine and watch one of your favorite funny movies while you're working out, or call a trusted friend or relative who is full of positive energy and will cheer you up.

If you're a Depressed Eater, you should:

- Avoid sweets to reduce blood sugar spikes.

- Select low glycemic index foods.

- Select fresh alternatives to processed foods.

- Remove "trigger foods" from the refrigerator and pantry.

- Keep some low-cal snacks around as to not be tempted by other items.

Glycemic Index: The glycemic index, or GI, measures how quickly a carbohydrate-containing food raises blood glucose. A food with a high GI raises blood glucose more than a food with a medium or low GI. Fat and fiber tend to lower the GI of a food. As a general rule, the more cooked or processed a food, the higher the GI.

Food for the Depressed Eater

HIGH-FIBER CARBOHYDRATES:
squash (acorn, butternut, winter), artichokes, leeks, lima beans, okra, pumpkin, sweet potatoes or yams, turnips, legumes (black lentils, adzuki beans, cow peas, chick peas, French beans, kidney beans, lentils, mung beans, navy beans, pinto beans, split peas, white beans, yellow beans), brown rice, quinoa, hummus, millet.

LOW GLYCEMIC INDEX FRUITS:
blackberries, blueberries, boysenberries, elderberries, raspberries, strawberries, sour green apples.

LEAN PROTEINS:
chicken or turkey breast, all fish, pork tenderloin, extra-lean ground beef or buffalo, shrimp, crab, beans, legumes.

Eating Strategies for the Depressed Eater

The Depressed Eater will need to develop some rules about where and when they eat. Many Depressed Eaters are "grazers" and tend to feed their emotions through-out the day, so it is important to create meal and snack times that fit into your schedule.

Examples of helpful rules include: no eating in bed, no eating in front of the TV or on the couch, always put a portion of food in a bowl or on a plate instead of eating from the package, and no eating standing in front of the refrigerator with the door open. These are good rules to model for your family, too! Begin with small changes like using smaller serving dishes so portions are better controlled and trying to avoid fatty and fried foods. If you currently eat fried food five times a week, try to cut down to two times, then one, and then only once or twice a month.

Meals should be at least four hours apart; if they are more than four hours apart, be sure to schedule a snack for yourself. Create a "meal experience" (a meal at which you set the table, light a candle, and enjoy your meal instead of rushing through it) or have a meal with family and friends at least twice a week. Many families tend to fend for themselves and eat on the go. If that is the case in your household, you can still create an experience for yourself. And if you live alone, inviting someone to share a meal with you (or hosting a potluck) can make your meal experience even more enjoyable.

Some Depressed Eaters may also benefit from identifying their "worst times." When are you most likely to depressed eat? Is it during the day when everyone is gone? At work? At night? Come up with alternative activities that you can participate in during your worst time—stretching, going on a short walk, reading, doing puzzles, anything to keep you busy.

Skinny Tips for the Depressed Eater

Drink an eight-ounce glass of water (ideally warm water with lemon) before each meal. Stay hydrated all day. Instead of consuming drinks with calories, try sparkling water or herbal tea.

Recipe for the Depressed Eater

Stir-fry recipes are great for the Depressed Eater because they're mostly vegetables so you can eat a good-sized portion. If you don't like to cook, you can find pre-cut vegetables to save on chopping time—or you can take the time to chop everything and make your meal preparation an activity that you enjoy.

Low-Carb Chicken, Broccoli & Mushroom Stir-Fry

PREP TIME: 15 minutes
COOK TIME: 15 minutes
SERVINGS: 4

Ingredients

1 pound (2 breasts) boneless skinless chicken breast, cut into 1-inch pieces
2 garlic cloves, finely chopped
2 teaspoons gingerroot, finely chopped
1 medium onion, cut into thin wedges
1 cup baby-cut carrots, cut in half lengthwise
1 cup chicken broth or stock
3 tablespoons low-sodium soy sauce
2 teaspoons sugar
2 cups broccoli flowerets
1 cup (3 oz.) sliced fresh mushrooms
1/2 cup red bell pepper, diced
2 teaspoons cornstarch

Instructions

Spray a 12-inch nonstick skillet with cooking spray; heat over medium-high heat. Add chicken, garlic, and gingerroot; stir-fry 2 to 3 minutes, or until chicken is brown.

Add onion, carrots, 3/4 cup of the broth, soy sauce, and sugar. Cover and cook over medium heat 5 minutes, stirring twice.

Add broccoli, mushrooms, and bell pepper. Cover and cook about 5 minutes more, stirring occasionally, until chicken is no longer pink in center and vegetables are crisp-tender.

Mix cornstarch with remaining 1/4 cup broth; stir into chicken mixture. Cook, stirring frequently, until sauce is thickened. Serve over steamed cabbage.

Nutritional Facts per serving:
  Calories 271
  Total Fat 5g
  Saturated Fat 1g
  Cholesterol 96mg
  Sodium 711mg
  Total Carbs 15g
  Dietary Fiber 3g
  Sugar 7g
  Protein 40g

Access a FREE download with more stir-fry recipes here: www.PsychedtobeSkinny.com

2

The Anxious Eater

The Anxious Eater eats due to anxiety about the present, past, or future. This is a person who has a hard time sitting still and will eat to calm the anxiety they are feeling. Anxious Eaters may be so wrapped up in their anxiety that they do not realize they are overeating; they often eat without knowing how much they are consuming. They may not even be totally cognizant of *what* they are eating.

Anxious Eaters are the ones at work or school who are always around the food or candy machine. The Anxious Eater usually eats quite quickly, taking little time to enjoy or savor their food. The Anxious Eater often multitasks while eating — working, running after their kids, or driving. Because the Anxious Eater is rarely present with their food, they tend to eat more and feel less satisfied than others when they are done with their meal.

Anxious Eaters need to learn to be present and put total focus on their food when eating so they can feel satisfied with what they have eaten. They need to learn to eat slowly and consciously enjoy their food.

If you're an Anxious Eater, you need to:

- Reduce stimuli while eating to reduce your anxiety.

- Facilitate identification of your anxiety issues.

- Review methods of coping in anxiety-provoking situations.

- Improve your stress management skills such as conscious muscle relaxation.

- Incorporate exercise into your routine to relieve your anxiety.

- Work on time management and prioritizing so you can make the time to have relaxed periods in which to eat.

- Vent your anxieties and fears to a therapist or trusted friend or relative.

- Know that this, too, shall pass.

- Participate in pleasant activities that may reduce your exposure to anxiety-provoking situations.

- Try to keep only healthy food around the house when you know you are going to be in anxiety-provoking situations.

Cognitive Behavioral Exercises for the Anxious Eater

Educate yourself on the impact of negative thinking and negative self-talk. Develop calming, positive self-talk and cognitive reappraisal. Use stress management techniques such as relaxation training, positive visualization (picturing yourself calm and anxiety-free), and breathing practices.

One great way to practice your breathing: Start by putting your right hand on your chest and your left hand on your abdomen. Inhale deeply through your nose or your mouth; really fill your lungs with air, and notice which hand raises more as you do so. If your right hand moves first you are a chest breather; if your left hand moves more you are a diaphragm breather. Inhale for three seconds and exhale for six seconds repeatedly—big, slow, relaxing breaths. If you're a chest breather, try to practice breathing through your diaphragm instead. It will make for a calmer, happier, healthier you. Breathe in. Breathe out. Don't you feel better already?

Stopping Negative Self-Talk

In order to develop healthy eating habits, you have to stop thinking negatively about your body and the food you put into it. Negative thoughts can cause high blood pressure, eating disorders, shingles, anxiety, depression, heart disease, stomach ulcers, acne, and more. Instead of letting your negative thoughts take over, use positive self-talk to stay mentally and physically healthy. You can do this in three simple steps.

Step 1:   Recognize Negative Self-Talk. When you think negative thoughts like: "I'm fat," "No one likes me," "I'll never amount to anything," "I'm a loser," or "I will never be happy," you bring about negative results and negative feelings toward yourself and others, trapping you in a cycle where people do avoid you—not because you're overweight, but because they want to be around positive people.

Step 2:   Set a New Mental Map of Positive Self-Talk. Consciously think positive thoughts like: "I will lose weight," "I will get that degree, good grade, or job," and "I have a lot going for me." Run through the good things you have going for you in your head. Tell yourself, "I will be and deserve to be happy."

Step 3:   Replace Old Thought Processes with Powerful New Ideas. Now that you have some practice thinking positive thoughts, take your old negative thoughts and turn them around: "I used to be fat and unhealthy, but now I will be healthy and thin"; "I was unhappy with my weight, but I will be happy with my new body soon"; "I used to have a hard time completing things, but now I will accomplish everything I set out to do"; "I used to not love myself, but I will love myself from now on"; "I never thought I was amazing before, but now I know I am an amazing person"; "I never thought people liked me, but now I know there are many people out there who love me."

It feels a lot better to make yourself feel good rather than bad, doesn't it? We believe in you—but you have to believe in you, too. Start practicing now!

Solution-Focused Exercises for the Anxious Eater

Picture in your mind your ideal situation. Consider, for instance, if when you felt anxious you practiced your breathing and meditative exercises and achieved a state of relaxation instead of reaching for food. Think of how good you would feel if you taught yourself to avoid unhealthy eating habits and established healthy eating habits—habits that, in turn, might lead to a healthier, more centered lifestyle.

Physical Exercise for the Anxious Eater

Like the Depressed Eater, the Anxious Eater should check with their medical doctor before they begin exercising to make sure their anxiety is not a medically-based issue such as mitral valve prolapse, hyperthyroidism, or hypertension. Be sure to let your medical doctor know if you are taking any psychiatric drugs or are using illicit street drugs.

For reducing generalized anxiety, as well as your proclivity for panic attacks, aerobic exercise is the key. What type of exercise you do depends on your fitness level. If you do not normally exercise, you may want to start out by taking brisk walks. If you are in good physical shape, you may enjoy running, cycling, swimming, hiking, or skiing, among other activities. Aerobic exercise requires sustained activity in your larger muscle groups, reduces skeletal muscle tension, and increases cardiovascular conditioning. Regular aerobic exercise has been shown to reduce stress and phobic reactions.

If socializing is important to you, team sports or group classes may be just what the doctor ordered. Try basketball, volleyball, hockey, football, aerobic dance, belly dancing, salsa dancing, kickboxing, or karate (which can also help center you). If the state of physiological arousal caused by rigorous exercise reminds you too much of the symptoms of panic or a panic attack and makes you feel self-conscious, you may want to start out walking by yourself or with a trusted friend or family member; you can gradually build up to running and other, more rigorous activities. If too much stimuli turns your workout into a panic situation, work out by yourself or in a quiet place. Remember to mix up your exercise regimen so you do not become bored and quit—this is a very important key to your mental health.

Lastly, you may want to incorporate some type of yoga into your exercise curriculum. There are many types of yoga, including heated yoga and yoga to tone. Yoga will help you to get the exercise you need, and it also incorporates helpful relaxation techniques. It is very important for anxiety-ridden individuals to remember to breathe, especially when nervous, and yoga will teach you to concentrate on your breath. Namaste, everyone.

If you're an Anxious Eater, you should:

- Plan meals at least a day in advance; a weekly plan is even better.

- Eat something within an hour of waking up.

- Limit your fast food intake, especially from drive-thrus.

- Keep a bottle of water with you at all times.

- Start a food journal.

Food for the Anxious Eater

NUTRIENT-DENSE FOODS:
kale*, watercress*, collard greens*, Swiss chard*, bok choy*, arugula*, romaine lettuce*, carrots, cabbage, cauliflower, broccoli, bell peppers, mushrooms.

HEALTHY FATS:
avocados, olives, olive oil, grapeseed oil, walnuts, almonds, pumpkin seeds.

FRESH, NUTRIENT-DENSE FRUITS:
strawberries, blackberries, raspberries, blueberries, pomegranates, cantaloupe.

*Most nutrient-dense options.

Eating Strategies for the Anxious Eater

The Anxious Eater's biggest challenge is to be *mindful* about eating. The frenzied rush and go-go-go mindset of Anxious Eaters makes meals whiz by in a blink. When eating, pause, then take a bite of food (just one bite—not as much as you can fit in your mouth), chew slower than usual, *taste* what you're eating, and swallow. Take a breath and pause before the next bite, and then repeat the steps above. While you're chewing, think about how the food tastes: Is it sweet, savory, sour, or salty? Is it cold, hot, or warm? How does it feel in your mouth? Is it mushy, soft, chewy, crunchy, or hard? When you do this, you will likely discover that many of your typical food choices don't actually taste very good—and that nutrient-dense and fresh foods, in contrast, have amazing flavor.

The "20-Minute Rule" is important for the Anxious Eater. It takes twenty minutes for your stomach to signal your brain that you are full. If you eat quickly or are often on the go and not paying attention to what you're putting in your mouth, it is common for your "satiety meter" to be skewed—especially if you have been eating this way for a number of years. You want to eat until you are *satisfied*—not too full, but not feeling hungry anymore either. If you tend to eat unmonitored quantities of food (a bag of potato chips while watching TV) or high-calorie, low-nutrition foods in a hurry (a double cheeseburger and large French fries while driving), or even if you usually take a second serving right after finishing your first, you have trained your satiety meter that *full* or *stuffed* equals *satisfied*. If you gobble down a double cheeseburger and fries in ten minutes, you have blown by satisfied and full and gone straight to feeling stuffed—and now your body thinks that you have to feel stuffed to feel satisfied.

SATISFIED ➤ FULL ➤ Stuffed

A great way to practice eating more slowly is to engage in a conversation when you eat with your friends or family so you are pausing to talk between bites of food. You can be the one to start a discussion—even something as easy as "What did you do yesterday?" or "Have you read any good books lately?" will spark conversation. People will almost always respond and then ask you the same question back. Remember your manners; don't talk with your mouth full! This will not help to slow you down.

Dining out is another way to practice eating slowly, even if you are dining by yourself. Most of us will instinctively eat a little more slowly at a restaurant because we don't want to look like we are shoveling food into our mouth when we're in public. You can also ask your server to stagger your courses so you don't get all of your food at once. Keep in mind that most restaurants are trying to "turn" their tables quickly—they want you in and out as fast as possible. Don't let them set the pace of your meal. You can order a salad to start and wait until you're done with it before ordering your entrée if you want to take things more slowly—and an added benefit of this approach is that you may realize that you don't want as much food as you originally thought because some time has passed since you started eating. Maybe you'll end up ordering a half entrée, or even just a cup of soup. If you are always on the run and doing things for others, choose one day a week to treat yourself to lunch and practice mindful eating.

Skinny Tips for the Anxious Eater

Try air-popped popcorn sprayed with low-calorie butter spray. It's a yummy option for those times that your anxiety makes you want to eat but you want to be healthy.

Drink herbal tea instead of eating when you're itching for a snack; cold or hot, it will fill you up and satisfy your craving for flavor.

Recipe for the Anxious Eater

Slow cooker recipes are ideal for the Anxious Eater who is often on the go. Throw a few things in your slow cooker in the morning, and by the time you get home, dinner is ready. This recipe is loaded with nutrients. Before adding the kale or spinach, you can freeze half the soup and save it for later (this is especially helpful if you are only cooking for one or two). You can add chicken or ground turkey as well, if desired.

Savory Bean & Spinach Soup

PREP TIME: 15 minutes
COOK TIME: 5–7 hours
SERVINGS: 6

Ingredients

32 oz. vegetable stock or broth
12 oz. water
1 15-oz. can tomato puree
1 15-oz. can small white beans or Great Northern
  beans, drained and rinsed
1/2 cup uncooked brown rice
1/2 cup finely chopped yellow onion
1 teaspoon dried basil
1/4 teaspoon sea salt
1/4 teaspoon black pepper
2 garlic cloves, chopped
8 cups coarsely chopped fresh spinach and/or kale
  leaves
Finely shredded Parmesan cheese, to taste (omit for
  dairy-free)

Instructions

In a 3-1/2- or 4-quart slow cooker, combine vegetable broth, water, tomato puree, beans, rice, onion, basil, salt, pepper, and garlic. Cover and cook on low-heat setting 5 to 7 hours or on high-heat setting 2-1/2 to 3-1/2 hours.

Just before serving, stir in spinach and/or kale and sprinkle with Parmesan cheese.

Nutrition Facts per serving:
Calories 198
Total Fat 1g
Saturated Fat 0g
Cholesterol 0mg
Sodium 336mg
Total Carbs 38g
Dietary Fiber 6g
Sugar 6g
Protein 10g

Access a FREE download with more slow cooker soup recipes here: www.PsychedtobeSkinny.com

3

The Situational Eater

The Situational Eater may eat to due to certain situations or circumstances—because there are stimuli around them that reminds them of times when they have been seduced or comforted by food. The Situational Eater may be your cruise boat eater—"We have to eat all the food that is served to us because it is free with the cruise"; they may be your buffet eater—"We have to eat all we can because we paid for this and we have to get our money's worth"; and they may be your vacation eaters—"We have to try all the local cuisine while we are here in Mexico." Situational Eaters are often called coach potatoes because they eat when they sit down to watch TV.

Situational Eaters are often the people who gain the most weight over the holidays. Christmas, Hanukah, Thanksgiving, New Year's Eve, and other events are all times to celebrate and rejoice with family and friends—and good food. Some Situational Eaters are stimulated by sports events as well (both on television or when watching the real thing). Sporting events are synony-mous with peanuts, pretzels, hotdogs, popcorn with lots of butter, and beer, after all—and have you ever seen healthy food run out first at a Super Bowl Party?

Some friends or relatives may trigger the Situational Eater, whether it's a friend or relative who likes to eat the same type of food or someone who they do not think will judge them if they overindulge. Being around food that they don't usually get to eat (fair food, for example, or just an unusual cuisine) often stimulates the Situational Eater as well.

The Situational Eater needs to be cognizant of *why* they are eating. They need to change their patterns—instead of eating when their impulse is triggered, they have to train themselves to do something else such as go for a walk or call a friend.

If you're a Situational Eater, you need to:

- Think about situations that do not involve food or eating; when have you had a good time when you were not consuming food?

- Think of some activities (like exercise) that make you feel better about yourself.

- Do something that requires focused concentra-tion, such as reading a good book or taking a class or course just for fun.

- Identify thoughts associated with your situa-tional eating. Figure out what thought process stimulates your eating.

- Identify who, where, when, and what triggers your situational eating.

- Ask yourself how you felt the last time you indulged in situational eating. What was your mood like before and after?

- Not let guilt or shame take control of your emotions after a situational eating binge; know that everyone has vices and loses control at times.

- Talk to a trusted friend or relative about your situational eating if you feel secretive about or ashamed of it.

- Forgive yourself after bouts of situational eating; know that you are working on acquiring the tools and skills to control your situational eating.

Cognitive Behavioral Exercises for the Situational Eater

Identify cognitive themes that promote your tendency to be a Situational Eater:

I situational eat when I am feeling

_____

_____

I situational eat when others are

_____

_____

I tend to situational eat most when the world is

_____

_____

After I situational eat, I feel

_____

_____

Access a FREE download of cognitive behavioral exercises for the Situational Eater here:
http://www.PsychedtobeSkinny.com

Solution-Focused Therapy for the Situational Eater

Picture what you really want for yourself. What would you like your life to look like? Imagine yourself in control over your situational eating, whether out with friends at a party or simply hanging by yourself. Imagine a happier, healthier, thinner you that is not feeling guilty or frustrated—a you that is happy about your lifestyle change and the fact that you have changed your physical and mental well-being for the better.

Physical Exercise for the Situational Eater

As with all people who find themselves unstable at times, it is of the utmost importance that the Situational Eater see their medical doctor to rule out any physical issues that maybe related to their state of mind before starting a new exercise regimen. Situational Eaters sometimes suffer from high blood pressure, high cholesterol, depression, or anxiety. If you are suffering from depression or anxiety, you may want to talk to your medical doctor or your psychiatrist about medication options. If you're on medication and wish to stop taking it, talk to your medical doctor or your psychiatrist first, as they will want you to slowly taper off any medication you have been on for any period of time.

At times the Situational Eater may find that they would rather exercise alone. This can take the form of running or exercising on the elliptical machine while watching TV at home. Depending on your mood, you may at times not want to exercise at all—but try to go for a walk or a short run, even if you're feeling gloomy. It is sure to help improve your mood. If you need something more interactive, Pilates is always a good choice, as is yoga, Zumba, volleyball, rock climbing, horseback riding—anything that keeps you focused and energized. Trying new things that require mental *and* physical stamina will advance your self-esteem, and it will give you something new to talk about over lunch. (You can really work up your interest factor when you're talking about your latest pole-dancing class.) Try advancing beyond your comfort level at times; it will pay off.

Lastly, keep a record of your daily activities. Include the date, time, type of exercise, and duration of the activity. Do this on a daily basis for one month. If you had planned to exercise and ended up not doing it, write the reason you were not able or ready to exercise. If you are feeling ill, of course, don't force yourself to work out. If you are finding yourself feeling bored with exercising solo, find a partner who is responsible and would like to exercise with you. If you do decide to find a workout partner, be sure to make it someone you trust and can have fun with.

If you're a Situational Eater, you should:

- Remove most "party" trigger foods from your pantry (i.e., chips, nuts, candy, ice cream).

- Look at your schedule at the beginning of each week to determine what events are coming up and try to plan an activity before or after the event so it isn't all about food.

- Write down a list of 10 to 15 healthy foods that you really love and keep them on hand.

- Avoid excessive alcohol intake at party situations; limit yourself to 2 drinks.

Food for the Situational Eater

LOW-FAT FOODS:
non-starchy vegetables* of all kinds, whole grains (including brown rice, quinoa, barley, oatmeal, whole grain/high fiber cereals), low-fat dairy.

HIGH-PROTEIN FOODS:
poultry, fish, egg whites, Greek yogurt, cottage cheese, lean beef and pork in moderation.

HIGH OMEGA-3 FOODS:
seafood (including halibut, herring, oysters, salmon, mackerel, sardines, trout, and fresh tuna), non-GMO tofu, flaxseed/flaxseed oil, walnuts, pumpkin seeds,

chia seeds, sesame seeds, cauliflower, soybeans, navy beans, kidney beans.

*Starchy vegetables include corn, peas, potatoes, and yams/sweet potatoes.

Eating Strategies for the Situational Eater

The Situational Eater often looks at "situations"—parties, gatherings, sporting events, dining out, and vacations—as "all or nothing" events, and they gravitate toward ALL. For example, a Situational Eater that is following some type of diet or healthier eating plan is likely to throw it all out the window while on vacation and indulge in drinks and desserts at every meal. This very often leads to increased guilt, as well as increased weight.

A good strategy for the Situation Eater is to look at trying new *healthy* foods as part of a splurge and the experience of an event (you could order a type of grilled fish you haven't eaten before, for example). Taking the edge off of your hunger prior to an event can also be helpful, and it is very easy to accomplish. Have a small snack—something around 100 calories—before every event. This could be a glass of milk (dairy, soy, almond, or coconut), a small yogurt, a handful of walnuts, celery with nut butter, or carrots and hummus. If you are not starving when you arrive to wherever you're headed, it will be easier for you to make healthier choices.

When you are at an event, mingle away from the buffet table and kitchen as this will prevent you from grazing on snack foods during conversation. Holding your beverage glass in your dominant hand can also help keep you from snacking because it makes it more awkward for you to pick up something to eat. When you do go over to a buffet, choose only five things, and take a moderate portion of each one—about half of a fistful—and don't go back for seconds. This will make you choose the foods that you really like and control the amount you consume, rather than having a few bites of a number of things (some of which you probably don't love) and then going back for seconds.

When it is time for dessert at an event, take "three polite bites,"—that's it. Savor the bites and enjoy the flavor. Limiting yourself to three bites will give you the satisfaction of having tried the dessert but not the extra calories and sugar rush you'd get if you overindulged.

Skinny Tips for the Situational Eater

Drink zero-calorie sparkling water with fresh lime, lemon, or cucumbers (spa water!) in it, or beverages sweetened with Stevia. Limit your consumption of sugar and artificial sweeteners.

Recipe for the Situational Eater

The Situational Eater needs to keep ingredients on hand for meals that are easy to throw together—this will prevent you from indulging in heavy snacking while preparing a meal. Soup, salad, and sandwich combinations are great options.

Greek Chicken Salad Pita Sandwich & Butternut Squash Soup

Both of these recipes can be made in advance to have on hand for several quick meals.

Sandwich

PREP TIME: 15 minutes
SERVINGS: 4

Ingredients

2 chicken breasts, cooked and diced
3 tablespoons extra-virgin olive oil
1 tablespoon red wine vinegar
2-3 plum/Roma tomatoes, seeded and chopped
1 cucumber, peeled, seeded, and diced
1 bell pepper (red, green, yellow, or orange), seeded
   and chopped
1/2 red onion, chopped
1/2 cup chopped fresh Italian parsley
1/2 cup crumbled feta cheese
4 whole-wheat pita breads (8-inch diameter), halved

Instructions

Whisk olive oil and red wine vinegar in large bowl; season with salt and pepper. Mix tomatoes, cucumber, bell pepper, red onion, and parsley into dressing. Stir in feta cheese.*

Using slotted spoon, transfer salad mixture to pita bread halves. Serve sandwiches immediately. (Serving size: 1/2 pita with approximately 1/2-cup of chicken salad.)

*Salad can be made two days ahead. Cover and chill.

Nutritional Facts per serving:
Calories 215.3
Total Fat 9g
Saturated Fat 3g
Cholesterol 32mg
Sodium 300mg
Total Carbs 21g
Dietary Fiber 3g
Sugar 2g
Protein 14g

Soup
PREP TIME: 15 minutes
COOK TIME: 25 minutes
SERVINGS: 6

Ingredients
2 tablespoons extra-virgin olive oil
1 carrot, diced
1 celery stalk, diced
2 shallots, diced
4 cups cubed butternut squash, fresh or frozen
1/2 teaspoon chopped fresh thyme
4 cups low-sodium chicken or vegetable stock
1/2 teaspoon fine sea salt
1/2 teaspoon ground black pepper

Instructions

Heat oil in a large soup pot. Add carrot, celery and onion; cook for 3 or 4 minutes, until onions begin to turn translucent.

Stir in butternut squash, thyme, chicken or vegetable stock, salt, and pepper. Bring to a boil, then reduce heat and simmer for about 30 minutes, until squash is fork-tender.

Let cool slightly, then puree soup in a food processor or blender in batches. Top with dollop of plain Greek yogurt if desired.

Nutritional Facts per serving:
Calories 145.2
Total Fat 6g
Saturated Fat 1g
Cholesterol 5mg
Sodium 438mg
Total Carbs 18g
Dietary Fiber 2g
Sugar 5g
Protein 5g

4

The Bored Eater

The Bored Eater eats due to that fact that they have nothing else to do; they lack a sense of sense of purpose or believe that they do. They grab a bag of chips, cookies, or a pint of ice cream because they need a distraction. The Bored Eater sees food as entertainment—as a way to keep them occupied—rather than as a nutritious substance for their body. Many Bored Eaters eat in their car while driving or at home while watching TV because they do not find whatever they're doing stimulating enough to hold their interest. Some Bored Eaters go out to eat in order to end their boredom, or eat at parties when they find the conversation lacking.

The Bored Eater may be a stay-at-home mom or dad who spends their days taking their children to football, soccer, basketball, hockey, or dance classes, cleaning the house, doing laundry, grocery shopping, and making meals while *Sesame Street, Dora the Explorer,* or *SpongeBob SquarePants* plays in the background for hours on end. Eating may be their way of escaping from their lack of stimuli; their environment does not stimulate them so they use food to combat their boredom. Some moms and dads will often eat while watching their children's sports practices or games for the same reason.

The Bored Eater may be an adult, teen, or child in a car, on a plane, or in the subway who eats to make the trip seem shorter; a kid who has to watch their sibling in a sports game or performance; or anyone who goes out to eat at a restaurant with people they find uninteresting, and who orders food or dessert to get through the boring meal.

If you're a Bored Eater, you need to:

- Figure out what you feel you are lacking in your personal life and try to find a way to fill that need.

- Journal about when you are bored eating to pinpoint the times you are most likely to do it.

- Try to find an alternate activity, like knitting or reading, when you're tempted to bored eat.

- Try to avoid places that you know cause you to bored eat.

- Find something else interesting to do besides bored eating when you're traveling or commuting, like listening to your favorite tunes or a book on tape.

- If you are bored eating in the evening due to lack of stimuli, get into the habit of going for a walk or bike ride with a friend around that time.

- Try to stimulate your senses another way when you're tempted to bored eat—with an e-reader, a computer, anything that keeps your mind occupied.

- Call a friend or relative who you can have a stimulating conversation with when you're feeling like you want to bored eat.

- Take some classes, do volunteer work, or enroll in a gym to keep busy.

- Remember to take care of your own needs and make sure your environment is stimulating for you so you can be healthy for yourself and your loved ones.

Cognitive Behavioral Exercises for the Bored Eater

Start a log to keep track of when you are bored eating. Put down the time of day and what you were doing at the time. Try to avoid environments and places that exacerbate your bored eating such as places with concession stands and food machines. Start a group with other Bored Eaters where you can band together to think of alternative means of entertainment; there are many Bored Eaters out there that would love to help and get help from other Bored Eaters!

Solution-Focused Exercises for the Bored Eater

Try to imagine yourself with a lifestyle that's healthy and guilt-free. What would that look like? Picture yourself doing healthy activities for yourself and your loved ones. Envision yourself getting ready to bored eat while watching television but instead getting up and going for a run or walk. See an image of a slimmer, healthier you that looks and feels amazing. Draw a picture of what you will look like when you are done bored eating; remember to put a smile on your face!

Physical Exercise for the Bored Eater

Check with your medical doctor before beginning a new exercise regimen, especially if your bored eating has led to significant weight gain, as you may have developed hypertension, type 2 diabetes, degenerative arthritis, or other physical ailments. A mental health provider can also help you decipher whether your eating is, in fact, bored eating and not depressive or anxious eating.

Physical exercise for the Bored Eater should be something that is mentally stimulating for them. The Bored Eater may want to take a snowboarding class or get involved with a large health club that can offer them many different forms of entertainment, from organized team sports like tennis, volleyball, or basketball to classes like spin cycling or water aerobics. If you're tight on cash, walking, bike-riding, cross-country skiing, or running may all be options. If you need more stimuli, invite a friend or relative to join you while you exercise. You should also mix up your exercise regimen to keep stimulated (studies show that people who perform different exercise routines from day to day work out longer and harder due to lack of boredom) and to help you work different muscle groups.

If you're a Bored Eater, you should:

- Drink one or two cups of caffeine-free herbal tea (hot or iced) daily.

- Avoid high-fat snack foods like potato chips, dips, nuts, cheese, cookies, and candy.

- Avoid high-calorie beverages like sodas, energy drinks, frozen coffee drinks, and fruit smoothies.

- Establish set meal times, eating every four to five hours with no snacking in between.

Food for the Bored Eater

COLORFUL FRUITS:
strawberries, raspberries, cherries, pomegranates, plums, blueberries, blackberries, purple grapes, apricots, cantaloupe, oranges.

COLORFUL VEGETABLES:
All dark leafy greens (spinach, kale, chard, collard greens, mustard greens), broccoli, brussels sprouts, eggplants, beets, tomatoes, bell peppers.

COLORFUL COMPLEX CARBOHYDRATES:
kidney beans, black beans, pinto beans, lentils, sweet potatoes, pumpkin, brown rice, red quinoa, buckwheat, whole/multi-grain bread, pumpernickel bread, dark rye bread.

Eating Strategies for the Bored Eater

The Bored Eater is very likely to eat the same thing over and over and to choose pre-packaged/processed foods and snacks. The lack of stimuli in their environment translates into meals that are lacking anything special, making it easy to overeat and/or to eat mindlessly.

A great strategy for the Bored Eater is to start learning how to cook, or—if you already know how—to brush up and improve upon your cooking skills. This will give you something interesting to do and it will make meals more enjoyable. You can spend the time that you've been spending watching TV and mindlessly eating preparing new, healthy recipes, learning what seasonings to use for different meats and vegetables, and maybe even taking a cooking class. You also may want to experiment with different aromatic spices—spices that have bold flavors and aromas as well as health benefits—in order to enhance the overall sensory experience of your food. These spices include: cumin, coriander, cardamom, turmeric, cinnamon, ginger, nutmeg, anise, cloves, chili powder, and fennel. Eating colorful foods can also help; it can make your plate look more appealing and taste better, and will help you to think more about what you are eating.

The Bored Eater should not snack or graze on foods except when they have to go more than six hours between meals (even then, the snack should only be eaten after three to four hours have passed; this allows your insulin levels to reset and balance your overall hormones). When you "graze" constantly, you never feel actual hunger, which can lead you to eat until you are too full rather than simply satisfied (see graphic for the Anxious Eater).

The Bored Eater may also need to implement a few

"rules" for eating to break their bad habits. Examples of this are: never eat in bed (or leaned back in a recliner); never eat or drink right out of the package—put the suggested serving size of the food you're eating on a plate or in a bowl (even do this for single serving foods); never eat right out of the refrigerator or cabinet with the door open (for example, you don't want to grab a handful of crackers out of a box and eat them while you stand there deciding what you want to eat); always eat breakfast; always have water (sparkling or flat) or unsweetened tea with meals; and always allow yourself to save leftovers instead of eating everything "so it doesn't go to waste."

Access our FREE "Herbs & Spices Guide" here: www.PsychedtobeSkinny.com

Skinny Tips for the Bored Eater

Bring healthy snacks with you—veggies, nuts, or fruits that are cut up and ready to eat—if you are going somewhere that might stimulate your bored eating. Enjoy a healthy Green Drink two hours before dinner—it's colorful, loaded with veggies, and low in calories.

Recipe for the Bored Eater

Since you are spending more time cooking, recipes that include preparing a spice blend or sauce in addition to the main entrée are a great choice—they'll make the food preparation process more enticing, and you can use these components for future meals!

Salmon with Aromatic Spice Rub

PREP TIME: 10 minutes
COOK TIME: 15 minutes
SERVINGS: 2

Ingredients

2 tablespoons fennel seed, toasted
1 tablespoon coriander seed, toasted
1 teaspoon tellicherry peppercorns
1 tablespoon pink Himalayan salt (coarse)
2 salmon filets (5-6 oz.) with skin removed
1 lemon, cut into wedges

Instructions

Preheat oven to 375 degrees.

Combine fennel, coriander, peppercorns, and salt in a spice grinder (or Magic Bullet or clean coffee bean grinder) to create Aromatic Spice Rub*. Rub mixture on both sides of salmon filets.

Place salmon in baking dish and place in oven; bake for 12-15 minutes, until salmon turns an opaque pink.

Serve with lemon wedges.

*This rub can also be used on chicken and pork.

Nutritional facts per serving:
Calories 207.5
Total Fat 9.2g
Saturated Fat 1.4g
Cholesterol 78mg
Sodium 186.8mg
Total Carbs 1.2g
Dietary Fiber 0.7g
Sugar 0.1g
Protein 28.4g

5

The Recently Dumped Eater

The Recently Dumped Eater eats due to the stress of a breakup. The Recently Dumped Eater tries to fill the void of loss of love and the feeling of rejection that accompanies it with something comforting: food. These individuals are often so distraught that they do not want to leave their house or apartment, and are feeling hopeless and helpless. The Recently Dumped Eater may have the attitude of *Who cares what I look like?* or *What does it matter if I gain twenty pounds?*, or they may look at overeating as a form of revenge. Maybe your former partner always tried to get you to go to the gym or try the latest fad diet or eat what they were eating. Now you can eat whatever and whenever you desire, no matter how fattening or unhealthy the food, without your former partner's critical eye watching you.

Some Recently Dumped Eaters are so hurt they intentionally try to gain weight so that no one will find them attractive—they don't want to have to worry about falling in love with someone and getting their heart crushed again. Food becomes their armor. Many Recently Dumped Eaters find comfort in eating with a trusted friend—sharing the story of their breakup over a tub of decadent ice cream, for example. They will begin to avoid going to restaurants or other people's houses to eat because they are feeling so down over their broken relationship that they do not want to socialize or expend the effort to look nice. Recently Dumped Eaters may not even feel like showering or getting out of their comfy pajamas or sweats for days.

If you're a Recently Dumped Eater and you exhibit the kind of behavior described above for more than a week or so, you should consider seeking therapy. You may need to go on an antidepressant to help you through your trauma. The best treatment combination is usually an antidepressant and therapy from a mental health provider. If you are under eighteen and are feeling suicidal, homicidal, or in danger of injuring yourself, you should tell a parent or guardian so they can seek help from a mental health professional on your behalf. If you're an adult who's experiencing any of these symptoms, you should check yourself into a psychiatric hospital so you can speak to a mental health provider and receive help.

If the Recently Dumped Eater's feelings of hopelessness and helplessness still exist after several weeks, they may have become a Depressed Eater. If this is true for you, you may want to go back to Chapter 1 and read or re-read about depressed eating.

If you're a Recently Dumped Eater, you need to:

- Know that this, too, shall pass.

- Understand that time truly does heal all wounds.

- Believe in yourself and in all the good things you have to offer.

- Write down ten of your best attributes and read them to yourself out loud every day.

- Count the blessings that you do have (good friends or a close family, perhaps?), be thankful for all the good things you have in your life, and try not to dwell on the things that you don't have.

- Try to get out of the house daily; getting up and getting dressed can help with the hurt and confusion of a breakup).

- Not look at the breakup as your fault; it takes two to make a relationship work.

- Keep faith in yourself; learn to love yourself before looking for your next significant other.

- Find something interesting that occupies your mind; maybe immerse yourself in a new class or group activity, something cognitively stimulating.

- Seek professional help if you're not feeling better after a couple of weeks.

Cognitive Behavioral Exercises for the Recently Dumped Eater

Define a special time of day that you are allowed to think about your ex—say from 1:00 to 2:00 p.m. daily. During that time you can think about your ex, and ideally journal about him or her. If you think about them outside of that predetermined time frame, stop and remind yourself that you've made a commitment to only think about them during the prescribed time. If you start thinking about eating while thinking about your ex, just keep journaling; even if you run out of things to say, you can simply write *I don't know what to write*. As long as you keep your pen moving, something will eventually pop into your head. Plan an activity that will help you keep your mind off your ex and off eating that you can engage in after your allotted time for thinking and writing about your ex is over.

Solution-Focused Exercises for the Recently Dumped Eater

If you had a fairy godmother that was granting you a wish that involved what you would look and act like if you ran into your ex three months from now, what would you wish for? Think about how you would want to feel and how you would want to portray yourself physically, mentally, and spiritually. Keep picturing the person you want to become in your mind; if you believe in yourself, you will become everything that you just envisioned, even without a fairy godmother there to make it happen for you.

Physical Exercise for the Recently Dumped Eater

Since the Recently Dumped Eater often exhibits many symptoms that are similar to those of the Depressed Eater, you should see a doctor to rule out medical issues before focusing on physical fitness. Hypertension is just one of the physical symptoms that could occur as a result of the stress caused by a breakup. You should also inform your medical doctor if you are feeling suicidal, homicidal, or are in danger of injuring yourself.

When the Recently Dumped Eater begins to exercise, they may want to start with something they are familiar with and are good at; the dissolution of a relationship can often have a negative impact on one's self-esteem, so it's important to be able to feel success in other realms of your life. Congratulate yourself, even for small achievements. If you could run five miles a day before but are only able to run one or two miles now, you can still celebrate the fact that you got out of the house and ran even though you didn't feel like running. If it helps to have a trusted friend to run or walk with, make sure you incorporate this into your workout routine.

The Recently Dumped Eater needs to build their self-esteem, and physical exercise is a great way to do it. When you're ready, try joining a team sport—not only will it help you get in shape, it will get you out of the house and interacting with new people. Fast-moving sports that require focus such as basketball, volleyball, soccer, and doubles tennis are perfect for keeping your mind off your ex. The Recently Dumped Eater may also thrive in exercise facilities that have a lot of action, lights, and music, since the extra stimuli will help them focus more on their surroundings and less on their ex.

You may want to keep yoga or Pilates practices to a minimum for the first couple of months after a breakup; in general, these sports are less stimulating and more relaxing, which can create too much space for thinking about your ex.

Access a FREE download of 5 Fast Exercises you can do at home here: www.PsychedtobeSkinny.com

If you're a Recently Dumped Eater, you should:

- Limit how often you pick up take-out food or have food delivered.

- Invite a friend over or to go out to dinner at least one time per week.

- Keep an online food and exercise diary that you can share with friends on social media so you have positive health interactions with others.

- Shop for produce two to three times per week, selecting only small quantities so it stays fresh.

- Avoid dairy products (milk, cheese, ice cream, yogurt, cottage cheese).

Food for the Recently Dumped Eater

HEALTHY FATS:
oils (olive, grapeseed, coconut), tree nuts (almonds, walnuts, cashews, hazelnuts), seeds (pumpkin, sunflower), olives, avocados.

LEAN MEATS:
chicken breasts, turkey breasts, bison/buffalo, pork tenderloin, tilapia, cod, halibut.

VEGAN PROTEINS:
dried beans/legumes (black-eyed peas, pinto beans, kidney beans, black beans, garbanzo beans, lentils), non-GMO tofu, and soybeans.

Eating Strategies for the Recently Dumped Eater

The Recently Dumped Eater should think about and then write down healthy foods/meals that they used to eat when they were single but gave up during their relationship. This will give them an opportunity to reset their mind and focus on what they like and what is healthy for their body.

Once you've made your list, clean out your pantry, refrigerator, and freezer so you can make a fresh start. This is not only a good opportunity to get healthier, it's an excuse to remove freezer-burned and old items (especially expired food) from your freezer and fridge. If there are foods left that are still good but are not on the list of foods you like after you're done, donate them to a local food pantry.

As you restock your groceries, be selective and try at least two new foods every week. Keep things that are easy and quick to prepare on hand so you won't be tempted to order in or pick up take-out. Take-out and delivery usually means pizza or Chinese food or something else that is high in fat—and it also means ending up with more than one serving, which can result in overeating (you will try to tell yourself that you are only going to eat two pieces of pizza, but let's be honest, we usually end up eating three or four!). Easy-to-prepare meals also can take your mind off of what it was like when you used to make dinner for two, or when your ex cooked for you. Remember, dinner doesn't have to be dinner food: you can have a bowl of cereal or scramble a couple of eggs and have them with a slice of whole-grain toast. Sandwiches are another easy go-to meal that are healthy and convenient.

The Recently Dumped Eater, like most, will benefit from eating more vegetables. Try to shop for fresh produce a few times a week; it will provide you with: (1) an activity; (2) an opportunity to try something new; and (3) increased nutrient availability for your body. Focus more on vegetables than fruit so you aren't over-eating fruit sugar, and go beyond lettuce, carrots, celery, and broccoli—try some less common low-calorie veggies like: arugula, beet greens, collard greens, kale, fennel, spaghetti squash, and Swiss chard. There are also some great complex carbohydrates—leeks, buckwheat, fingerling potatoes, and quinoa—that you may find new and interesting.

The Recently Dumped Eater should avoid dairy because many dairy products, especially cheese and ice cream, are high-calorie, comfort/overindulgence foods. You will be able to add dairy back into your diet in a few months, once you have established your new food palate, but initially you should steer clear of it. You'll also want to limit your alcohol intake; alcohol is a depressant, and may cause you to think about or obsess over your ex (all the while adding extra calories to your diet!). Think about the previous question we had you ask yourself: Whom do you want to be if you run into your ex three months from now? Odds are you don't want to be the intoxicated party animal that has gained weight. Instead, imagine a healthier you with glowing skin and a clear mind, all from better nutrition and mental habits.

Skinny Tips for the Dumped Eater

Don't think or talk about your ex before or during your meal, and don't go to the restaurants you used to go to with your ex—the emotional distress it causes may lead you to eat more and make unhealthy choices. At home, treat yourself in small ways: eat off of pretty plates, even if you're just having a quick sandwich, and drink out of a beautiful wine glass, even if you're just drinking sparkling water.

Recipe for the Recently Dumped Eater

Fast and easy meals generally don't require recipes; it's just a matter of having basic ingredients around for sandwiches, or chicken breasts (which you can buy already cooked and frozen), bagged salad mixes, and the like. This easy frittata recipe is something you could quickly make for dinner and then have for breakfast over the next couple of days.

Slow Cooker Vegetable Casserole

PREP TIME: 20 minutes
COOK TIME: 4-6 hours (low) or 2–2-1/2 hours
(high), stand 5 minutes
SERVINGS: 8

Ingredients

19-oz. can cannellini or pinto beans (low sodium)
19-oz. can garbanzo or fava beans (low sodium)
1/4 cup purchased basil pesto, divided
1 medium onion, chopped
4 cloves garlic, minced
1 1/2 teaspoons dried Italian seasoning, crushed
1 package cooked plain polenta, cut in 1/2-inch-
thick slices
2 tomatoes, thinly sliced
3 cups fresh greens for wilted salad
(choose one or a combination: spinach, arugula,
chard, radicchio)

Instructions

Rinse and drain beans. In large bowl combine beans, 2
tablespoons of pesto, onion, garlic, and Italian seasoning.

In 4 to 5-quart slow cooker, layer half of bean mixture,
half of polenta; add remaining beans and polenta. Cover;
cook on low heat setting 4 to 6 hours or on high heat setting 2 to 2-1/2 hours.

Add tomato and greens. Combine remaining pesto and 1 tablespoon of water. Drizzle pesto mixture on casserole. Let stand, uncovered, 5 minutes.

Nutritional Facts per serving:
Calories 270
Total Fat 6g
Saturated Fat 2g
Cholesterol 6mg
Sodium 440g
Total Carbs 46g
Dietary Fiber 10g
Sugar 8g
Protein 14g

6

The Fat is My Shelter Eater

The Fat is My Shelter Eater eats because their weight is a defense mechanism. These individuals are often sensitive and may be scared of being hurt by others, usually because they have been hurt in the past. They use their fat as a shield that protects them from having to deal with social situations and dating. Some Fat is My Shelter Eaters have a difficult time even leaving the house—some may even become agoraphobic (develop an abnormal fear of being in crowds, public places, or open areas) due to their weight. If this is true for you, you should contact a therapist as soon as possible.

Some Fat is My Shelter Eaters use their weight as an excuse not to have sex with their significant other. Some are presently or have been victims of sexual abuse, and they eat in the hopes that their weight gain will turn off their abuser, or use their weight as a shield against sex in an attempt to avoid having to relive painful memories of their abuse— they want people to see them as a non-sexual being so they can avoid being hurt, both mentally and physically.

Some Fat is My Shelter Eaters have gone through some sort of trauma—the death of a loved one, the loss of a job, or a natural disaster—and because of their resulting depression or grief, they use their fat as a way to isolate themselves. These types of Fat is My Shelter Eaters don't want to let others get too close to them so they won't have to worry about letting others know they are depressed, anxious, angry, dysthymic (suffering from low-grade yet continual depression), or hurt.

Fat is My Shelter Eaters will often say they don't want to go out because people will laugh at them or make fun of them for being overweight, or because they have nothing to wear that fits them. Many Fat is My Shelter Eaters don't like to go out to eat because they think they are being judged—they'll often say that they can tell that people are watching them the whole time they are eating. They may also use their weight to avoid going on vacations or traveling for work, saying that people don't want to sit near them because they are overweight. Warm-weather vacations or work destinations can be hard on Fat is My Shelter Eaters because they may be expected to go to the beach or wear less clothing than usual, which can cause them physical and emotional discomfort.

Fat is My Shelter Eaters will generally try to get out of workout-related activities, convinced that people will judge and ridicule them if they see them riding a bike, running, or playing a sport. Being in a gym, being around others who are working out, or doing anything that requires physical exertion—even something like going up and down the stairs at work—may be an emotional experience for the Fat is My Shelter Eater as they may think others are judging their labored breathing and large stature.

Fat is My Shelter Eaters will often avoid clothes shopping because they dislike going to the mall or public places where clothing is sold—and because of this, they often use the fact that they have no clothes to wear as a reason they can't go out of the house. Sometimes they will also hold on to the clothes they wore before they gained weight and refuse to buy any clothes in a larger size, insisting that they will eventually fit back into their old clothes.

If you are a Fat is My Shelter Eater and you are self-isolating and depressed—or if you know someone who exhibits these traits—please seek professional assessment of your mental state.

If you're a Fat is My Shelter Eater, you need to:

- Find out what your underlying issues are, either by self-reflection or undergoing psychoanalysis; Fat is My Shelter Eaters have deeper-seated issues than a love for food, and it's important to identify them.

- Journal every day about when and what you've eaten.

- Work to get in touch with your feelings and emotions.

- Go to a support group where other Fat is My Shelter Eaters are experiencing similar actions and reactions.

- Talk to a trusted friend or relative about why you feel the need to shelter yourself with weight.

- Work on self-love.

- Put time and attention into your personal hygiene and self-care, even if you don't feel like it.

- Volunteer for something that you have a passion for—helping others will make you feel happier.

- Get a physical from your medical doctor, and tell him or her about any feelings you have about your physical and mental health.

Cognitive Behavioral Exercises for the Fat is My Shelter Eater

Begin verbalizing and thinking about positive associations with healthy foods so you can eliminate your negative food-behavior mindset. Instead of saying or thinking "I always crave sweets when I've had a busy day," try "When I nourish my body with fresh, wholesome foods throughout a busy day I feel more productive." Instead of "I have to eat a big bowl of cereal or a bowl of ice cream right before I go to bed or I can't sleep," try "I'm going to enjoy a cup of hot chamomile tea before bed so that I can be relaxed and sleep well." The more you tell yourself "always" or "never" about a less healthy food, the harder it will be to change your habits.

Every time you have a desire or need to eat, write about how you're feeling first:

What am I feeling?

_____

_____

Am I really hungry or am I eating for another reason?

_____

_____

How am I going to feel after I eat this?

_____

_____

How can I soothe myself without eating?

_____

_____

What are five things that I love about myself?

_____

_____

Why am I using food to isolate myself from society?

_____

_____

Access a FREE download of cognitive behavioral exercises for the Fat is My Shelter Eater here:
http://www.PsychedtobeSkinny.com

Solution-Focused Exercises for the Fat is My Shelter Eater

If you could wake up in the morning and be exactly who you wanted to be, what would you look and act like? Would you have your ideal job? Would you have more money? Would you be in shape and proud of your body? Would you feel confident about going out in public? Would you laugh more? Would you be more physically active? Would people turn and look at you, not because of your weight but because you are fit and self-assured? Would you want to be social just so people could see how amazing you are? You can have all of the above. Have faith, love, and trust in yourself. Visualize all of these things coming true for you. You will amaze yourself and inspire everyone around you. You can and will make a difference in this world—you just have to believe in you.

Physical Exercise for the Fat is My Shelter Eater

First and foremost, check with your medical doctor before starting any new exercise routine. Weight gain can cause or be caused by hypertension, type 2 diabetes, degenerative arthritis, hypothyroidism, high blood pressure, and high cholesterol as well as psychological issues such as depression, anxiety, post-traumatic stress disorder, and low self-esteem. If your unhealthy eating habits are related to a psychological problem and you feel you need medication, talk to your medical doctor about this and see if he or she will prescribe you something or refer you to a psychiatrist. Keep in mind that the best recipe for success is a combination of prescribed psychiatric medication and therapy.

Since one of the behaviors common to the Fat is My Shelter Eater is trying to stay away from people, you will most likely be more comfortable exercising in your own home or yard—at least until you feel comfortable enough to exercise in front of others. If you cannot afford a personal trainer or personal exercise equipment, you can always use a workout video. If you have a second story in your house, climbing stairs is also a good form of exercise. Walks around the neighborhood are always a good idea. If you have young children, engage in more physical activities with them (even just chasing them around the house is fun exercise for you and for them). If you have a basketball hoop outside, a nice game of basketball with your family or with close friends is a great workout. If you are a couch potato, only let yourself watch television while you are working out in some way—possibly with a kettle bell or some small weights. If you have an outdoor bike but would rather not be riding it out in public, you can buy a stand for it that will allow you to ride it in the comfort of your own home (and it's much more affordable to do this than it is to buy a stationary bike). If you have a family member or friend who you trust and feel comfortable with, try to make some workout dates with them so you can get some social interaction alongside your physical activity.

Remember to start out slow in your workouts; even as you begin to shed some of your extra pounds, you may have some unconscious or conscious psychological issues that need to be addressed. As you begin to exercise more, you should be working on yourself mentally as well—with a therapist and psychiatric meds, if necessary. If you have been raped or sexually abused, please keep in mind that hypnosis, even by a professional, is highly unreliable and not recommended.

If you're a Fat is My Shelter Eater, you should:

- Put your scale in a closet and not weigh yourself for at least thirty days.

- Always make a grocery list when you go to the story, even you're only getting a few items, and stick to it.

- Consider adding a good multi-vitamin or other nutritional supplement to your daily routine.

- Beware of fad diets and things that sound too good to be true.

Food for the Fat is My Shelter Eater

FRUITS:
3 servings/day; 1 serving = 1/2 cup or 1 medium piece.

VEGETABLES:
Minimum 5 servings/day; 1 serving = 1 cup raw or 1/2 cup cooked.

WHOLE GRAINS/STARCHES:
4 to 6 servings/day; 1 serving = 1 slice bread or 1/2 cup starch.

DAIRY:
2 servings/day; 1 serving = 1 cup.

PROTEIN:
8 to 10 ounces/day; 1 serving = 3 ounces.

FATS & OILS:
5 teaspoons/day.

Serving Size References:

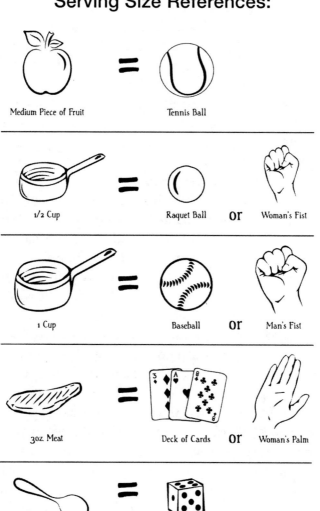

Medium Piece of Fruit	Tennis Ball		
1/2 Cup	Raquet Ball	or	Woman's Fist
1 Cup	Baseball	or	Man's Fist
3oz. Meat	Deck of Cards	or	Woman's Palm
1 tsp	1 Die		

Eating Strategies for the Fat is My Shelter Eater

One of the most important concepts to embrace for the Fat is My Shelter Eater is to focus on their *health*, not their weight. You can still be nourishing your body in a healthy manner, learning healthy behaviors, and changing your mindset before you start to see the scale move. When you are eating healthier your energy level will improve and you will be able to be more physically active; your mental clarity will improve; and you will be able to make consistent, healthier choices.

The Fat is My Shelter Eater needs to get back to the basics. Ultimately you will probably want to lose weight for health and self-esteem reasons, so it is important for you to learn what you are eating. Calories do matter — if you eat more calories than you burn you will gain weight — and if you have been eating without much thought, you probably haven't been paying attention to how many calories are in the foods that you eat. Start by looking at the food labels of the food items you commonly eat as well as what size portions you are eating. You can't lose weight if you overeat, regardless of the healthfulness of the foods you're eating.

You need to develop an awareness of everything you consume so you can learn how to enjoy all the foods that are part of a healthy diet. To start, add a zero to your current weight; this will give you a rough estimate, a baseline, of how many calories you can have each day. If you weigh 195 pounds, then 1,950 calories is around how many total calories you should have per day.

Now that you have your number, look at a nutrition label — premium ice cream, for example. A half-cup serving of ice cream contains 250-300 calories; there are four servings in a pint, so if you eat the entire pint, that's 1,000 to 1,200 calories—over half of your daily intake! You don't have to count calories; you just need start learning what's in the things you're eating. As time goes on, you will gradually learn to make better choices.

Skinny Tips for Fat is My Shelter Eater

Use smaller plates and bowls for meals so your portion sizes are more appropriate. Drink at least 80 ounces (approximately 2.5 liters) of low-calorie fluids daily (water, sparkling water, vegetable broth, herbal tea) throughout the day to give yourself a feeling of fullness.

Recipe for the Fat is My Shelter Eater

As you learn more about how many calories are in the foods you typically eat, you will want to look for lower-calorie alternatives to some of your favorite meals so you feel less deprived. Substituting ground turkey for ground beef in your burgers is an easy and great-tasting switch.

Zucchini Lime Turkey Burger

Staying with a basic nutrition program is easy when you heat healthier versions of familiar foods. Serve this turkey burger without a bun and with a side of organic black beans and green salad.

PREP TIME: 15 minutes
COOK TIME: 10 minutes
SERVINGS: 4

Ingredients

1 pound ground turkey breast
1 cup grated zucchini
2 tablespoons fresh chives, chopped finely
Juice of one lime
2 cloves garlic, minced
2 tablespoons sweet yellow onion, minced
1/2 teaspoon salt
1/2 teaspoon pepper
Cooking spray

Instructions

In large bowl, combine all ingredients. Form into four patties and place on plate. Refrigerate for at least one hour.

Heat grill pan over medium-high heat and spray with cooking spray. Place patties on pan and cook on each side until done (about 8 to 10 minutes total).

Nutrition Facts per serving:
Calories 182.6
Total Fat 9.6g
Saturated Fat 2.5g
Cholesterol 83.8mg
Sodium 372mg
Total Carbs 2.9g
Dietary Fiber 0.5g
Sugar 1.2g
Protein 21.8g

7

The Period Eater

The Period Eater has two elements that accompany their period: a physical one and a psychological one.

On the physical side, the Period Eater may crave foods because loss of blood has depleted her body of certain nutrients and vitamins. Loss of blood may especially lead the Period Eater to crave foods that are high in protein, sugar, and fat. The Period Eater often craves salt as well. Some Period Eaters describe this as Binge Period Eating—they say that once they get started on eating something that their body is craving they are unable to stop, even when they are feeling full. Some women state that they crave these foods the most a week before their period; this is when the body is hormonally imbalanced.

Psychologically, Period Eaters are often feeling depressed or anxious—or both—due to the hormonal changes occurring in their body. The Period Eater will frequently feel angry or frustrated with small things, and will fight with significant others, friends, or family members during this time, which only increases their anxiety and depression. The Period Eater is often able to abstain from foods that are high in fat, sugar, and salt until they have their period; it may be only when they have their period and are experiencing undue levels of anxiety and depression that they lose control over their normally healthy eating patterns.

The Period Eater is often tired due to the hormonal imbalance and blood loss prior to and during their period, so rather than engaging in any physical activity they may be more tempted to curl up on the couch with a bag of chips to watch television. Once this behavior begins, they can fall into a guilty spiral of lack of activity and eating unhealthy foods. Feeling bloated and heavier in body weight than normal can lead Period Eaters to feel guilty and depressed, even if they know that their cravings and binge-type eating will only last for a small amount of time, which only leads to more unhealthy eating behaviors.

It should be noted that between 3 percent and 8 percent of women have PMDD (Premenstrual Dysphoric Disorder), a condition that can cause severe anxiety, panic attacks, problems sleeping, mood swings that involve sadness or crying episodes, feelings of being out of control, feelings of hopelessness and helplessness and possible suicidal ideation, problems concentrating, disinterest in daily activities or relationships, and persistent irritability that affects others. These symptoms can be made worse by being overweight, having relatives with a history of PMDD, lack of exercise, drinking large amounts of caffeinated beverages, and alcohol abuse.

If you have PMDD, you need to:

- Get regular exercise during the month to lessen the severity of your symptoms.

- Try changing your sleeping habits—or if you suffer from severe insomnia, talk to your doctor about taking an over-the-counter sleeping pill while menstruating.

- Look into taking an antidepressant if depression is affecting your daily life.

- Look into temporarily using diuretics to reduce your fluid retention (though you should be sure to discontinue the diuretics after your period; long-term use of diuretics could be dangerous to your health).

- Use pain relievers such as ibuprofen or aspirin to ease back pain, cramping, or headaches.

- Talk to your doctor about the possibility of using a medication that suppresses ovulation, such as Depo-Lupron.

- Try cognitive behavioral therapy with a therapist once a month, during your period.

- Keep a diary of symptoms and when they occur.

If you're a Period Eater, you need to:

- Know that this, too, shall pass; this unhealthy eating is temporary.

- Get checked out by your medical doctor if you feel your periods are severe; if you have PMDD, your medical doctor may want to put you on an antidepressant.

- Get as much sleep and rest as possible, and recognize when your body needs more rest than usual.

- Take a deep breath and count to ten if you feel as if you may get angry over something that is not worth fighting about.

- Give yourself a break; you can splurge on your cravings once in a while and still maintain a healthy weight and lifestyle.

- Try to get in some exercise, even if that means simply taking the stairs instead of the elevator or parking your car far away from class or work so you are forced to walk farther than you normally would.

- Talk to a trusted friend, family member, or therapist if depression and/or anxiety are getting you down.

- Know that bloating is a normal part of having your period, and that it is a temporary phase. Wear something comfortable if you're feeling heavy and unattractive in your usual clothes, and remind yourself that you will be rockin' your skinny jeans in no time.

Cognitive Behavioral Exercises for the Period Eater

Track the times you have the most cravings and eat the most food. Is it a week before your period? The week of? Both? You should also track your emotions: When are your feelings the strongest? Are there certain times during your period when you feel less in control of your emotions than usual? Are there certain times during your period that you feel more angered, agitated, or irritated by others? Do you isolate more than usual when you have your period? Are you more tired than usual? Do you feel sluggish and less able to function physically and cognitively? Do you feel less attractive because of hormonal breakouts and hormonal bloating? Keep a journal that answers the questions stated above so you are better able to understand how your hormones are affecting your emotions and eating habits.

Solution-Focused Exercises for the Period Eater

If you could have the perfect week while still having your period, what would you envision? Would your cravings decrease to a manageable level? Would you be less grouchy and irritated? Would you have less bloating and fatigue? Would you be able to replace the unhealthy foods you were craving with healthy foods? Would you experience less cramping and discomfort? Through diet and exercise, all of this is possible. It may take a little bit more willpower, but you have the ability to live a happy and healthy life, even when you're having your period. Have faith in yourself and you will see yourself transform into a healthy, happy Period Eater.

Physical Exercise for the Period Eater

Before exercising, check with your medical doctor to make sure you are not dealing with any physical issues that could endanger your health. If you have PMDD, your periods are more severe than is normally seen with the premenstrual system, your medical doctor may want you to take special precautions during your period (they may want to put you on birth control to lesson your blood flow during your period, for instance).

If you experience cramping during your period, remember that exercise will help ease the pain. Put on your favorite songs and dance around your house; it's hard to be crabby when you're dancing and singing to music you love—who knows, you may just get in the mood to call a couple of friends and go out dancing to blow off some steam. You can also try walking on the treadmill while watching your favorite funny movie or biking to some good tunes; this will get your serotonin level up, which will make you feel better both mentally and physically. Call a friend or family member who makes you laugh and see if they would like to go for a walk or a run outside—or, if you have a dog, take your dog for a walk or to a dog park. Or how about doing aerobics to some old songs that remind you of high school or grade school, or challenging someone to a playful one-on-one game of basketball, hockey, Ping-Pong, volleyball, or any other sport you enjoy? Any physical activity you engage in is sure to lift your spirits.

If you're a Period Eater, you should:

- Eat a balanced diet and have little or no caffeine, sugar, salt, or alcohol during the time of your period or in the three to eleven days prior to it, as this is the time when your hormones are the strongest.

- Try nutritional supplements like magnesium, calcium, Vitamin D, and B6.

- Allow yourself to eat some of the food that your body is craving, but only in very small portions; don't overeat.

- Not let being on your period be an excuse for making poor food choices.

Food for the Period Eater

GLUTEN-FREE COMPLEX CARBOHYDRATES:
potatoes, sweet potatoes, rice, brown rice, buckwheat, dried beans and peas, lentils, quinoa, amaranth, winter squash.

DAIRY-FREE & SOY-FREE PROTEINS:
lean meats (fish, chicken, turkey, beef, pork), nuts and seeds (including nut butters), almond milk, rice milk, coconut milk (unsweetened).

SOY-FREE OILS & OTHER PRODUCTS:
olive oil, grapeseed oil, coconut oil, Bragg Liquid Aminos (substitute for soy sauce), other soy-free products.

Eating Strategies for the Period Eater

The Period Eater's meal problems are centered around hormones, and there are certain foods that may exacerbate hormonal problems or other digestive issues. Gluten, dairy, and soy are common allergenic foods that may cause your body to enter into an inflammatory state that can make your period symptoms even worse. If you're someone who experiences migraines or cluster headaches during your period, you'll also want to avoid these foods: alcohol (especially beer and red wine), chocolate, aspartame, excessive caffeine, aged or fermented cheeses (including cheddar, blue, Brie, and all hard and "moldy" cheeses), soy foods, nuts, citrus fruits, vinegar (both red and balsamic), nitrites (found in cured meat products like sausage, bacon, and hot dogs), sulfites (found in dried fruit and wine), MSG, yeast extracts, and hydrolyzed proteins.

Two important hormones to consider for the Period Eater are leptin and ghrelin. These hormones are specifically related to sleep and appetite and can play a role in food cravings.

Leptin is a satiety-promoting hormone that you release when you sleep; ghrelin, considered the counterpart of leptin, is a hormone that stimulates your appetite. When you are sleep-deprived (getting less than seven hours of sleep a night) your leptin levels decrease and your ghrelin levels increase, which means you will experience more hunger during the day. It is better for Period Eaters to get a good night's sleep, then, than it is for them to take naps during the day. Regular meal timing—making sure that you wait three to four hours between eating—can also help you keep your hormones in balance.

Skinny Tips for the Period Eater

Ease a chocolate-before-bed snack craving by heating up unsweetened chocolate almond milk; it is very low in calories, and the taste and warmth may help calm your mind. Make ice cubes or homemade popsicles out of equal parts of blended strawberries and water; pour sparkling water over the ice cubes for a refreshing drink.

Recipe for the Period Eater

Eating gluten and dairy free can be a challenge, but there are many ways to substitute foods and try new things. The recipe below, which uses Portabella mushrooms to create an open-faced "burger," is just one example of the variety of creative recipes out there.

Open-Faced Chicken & Pepper Sandwich

PREP TIME: 15 minutes
COOK TIME: 15 minutes
SERVINGS: 2

Ingredients
1 large boneless skinless chicken breast cut in thin,
    2-inch strips
Juice of 1 lemon
2 cloves garlic, minced
4 Portabella mushrooms, stemmed
2 teaspoons olive oil, divided
1/4 teaspoon sea salt
1/2 teaspoon fresh ground pepper
1/2 red or yellow bell pepper, sliced
1/2 green bell pepper, sliced
1/2 yellow onion, sliced
1/2 teaspoon dried basil

Instructions
Place chicken breast strips in medium bowl, then add
lemon juice and garlic. Stir.

Preheat oven to broil. Line a rimmed baking sheet with
foil and place mushrooms upside down (flat side up) on
top of foil. Brush with olive oil and sprinkle with salt
and pepper.

Place in oven and broil for 4 to 5 minutes on each side, until tender.

While mushrooms are broiling, heat a large skillet to medium-high heat. Sautee peppers and onions in olive oil for 2 to 3 minutes. Add chicken and basil and continue to cook until done, about 6 minutes.

Remove mushrooms from oven and place on plate. Using a slotted spoon or tongs, place equal amounts of chicken and pepper mixture on each mushroom half.

Nutrition Facts per serving:
Calories 204.4
Total Fat 6.8g
Saturated Fat 0.8g
Cholesterol 60mg
Sodium 543.8mg
Total Carbs 13.4g
Dietary Fiber 4.2g
Sugar 7.5g
Protein 27.6g

Download more FREE gluten- and dairy-free recipes here: http://www.PsychedtobeSkinny.com

8

The Peer Pressure Eater

This is the eater that eats when others around them are eating. The Peer Pressure Eater may eat because others say things to them like, "Oh come on, you can have a few nachos or French fries" or "Is that all you are going to eat? You can usually eat twice as many pancakes as that." Peer Pressure Eaters are often people who grew up in homes where everyone ate large portions of food and they felt as if they were expected to eat as much as the rest of the family. Mom, Dad, or Grandma would make large quantities of food for the family meal and encourage everyone to finish it all ("What am I going to do with all these leftovers?"), and the Peer Pressure Eater would end up eating more than they intended to.

Peer Pressure Eaters often feel large amounts of guilt after eating more than they anticipated. These are the folks who tell themselves that they won't eat large amounts of food or will eat something healthy but who feel a lack of control when they are around others who enjoy eating. These individuals may be fine eating on their own, but are incapable of saying "no" when other people tell them to eat more food or finish their plate before they leave the table.

It should not be overlooked that Peer Pressure Eaters often have low self-esteem. They want to be part of the group; they want to be accepted by the people pressuring them. The Peer Pressure Eater tends to seek out other Peer Pressure Eaters for moral support and eating binges. The more they eat, the more they isolate due to their weight gain, which keeps them stuck in their unhealthy cycle. They may not want to be around people who are not Peer Pressure Eaters, because being around people who they see as fit and skinny makes them feel even worse about themselves.

If you're a Peer Pressure Eater, you need to:

- Find other activities to do with your Peer Pressure Eater peeps, like biking or rollerblading.

- Learn to become more assertive. (If you are having trouble with this, talk to your therapist.)

- Try to stay away from places where Peer Pressure Eating is likely to occur.

- Learn to say "no thank you" to unhealthy choices.

- Learn to say "no" to second or third helpings.

- Try eating from a smaller plate or bowl, and encourage your Peer Pressure peeps to do the same.

- Work on self-esteem issues. Why are you having a hard time saying "no"? Seek out help from a therapist, if necessary.

- Take control of your eating—it is, after all, *your* body.

- If your family members are Peer Pressure Eaters, let them know that you would like to stick with your own meal plan.

Cognitive Behavioral Exercises for the Peer Pressure Eater

Journal about the times you eat the most and who is around when you do. Work on your self-esteem and your ability to say "no thank you" or "I would rather order something healthy off the menu." Try doing activities with your Peer Pressure peeps other than eating; something active like a hip-hop class or ice-skating. If your Peer Pressure peeps are in your family, you may want to join a group therapy session with other Peer Pressure Eaters and talk about your emotions. How was it to grow up in a Peer Pressure Eater family? I guarantee there will be others in your group who will understand how you feel.

Solution-Focused Exercises for the Peer Pressure Eater

If you were to daydream about the perfect you, how would you see yourself? Would you be in control of your weight and your food intake? Would your self-esteem and self-confidence be at an all-time high? Would you be more active? Would you be more respectful to your body and make healthier food choices? If a Peer Pressure Eater tried to get you to eat more than you wanted to, would you have the self-control and self-confidence to say "no"? This can be your reality: remember, the key is that you are in control of your body and your destiny. You can be self-assertive, confident, and healthy in your food choices and in life. We have faith in you—now have faith in yourself!

Physical Exercise for the Peer Pressure Eater

If you are a Peer Pressure Eater your weight probably fluctuates according to how often you are hanging out with other Peer Pressure Eaters. Peer Pressure Eaters especially tend to gain weight during the holiday season, as this is the time when people get together over food and alcohol. Before beginning a new exercise regimen, be sure to rule out anything physical that would cause you to gain and lose weight on a periodic basis, such as water retention or depression. If you are suffering from depression, make this known to your medical doctor; they will want to assess you for suicidal ideation, and may recommend that you see a therapist or try a SSRI or other antidepressant prescribed by your therapist.

Because Peer Pressure Eaters generally have low self-esteem, they may want to begin by engaging in physical activities that they are familiar with, and by starting out slowly in their workouts if they are not used to working out. Going for a walk around the block may be all the Peer Pressure Eater can do the first few days; eventually, however, they may want to start running (at a slow pace until they feel fit enough to pick up the speed). Biking is often a good sport for the Peer Pressure Eater as well because it allows you to burn a lot of calories in a short period of time. Whether you like to bike in a fitness class in the health club, bike alone in the gym, or bike outside, you are sure to shed some pounds if you bike while watching your weight and not Peer Pressure Eating.

If you are a Peer Pressure Eater and would like to join a team sport, try something that you feel confident in—a sport that will help your build your self-esteem. Maybe basketball, soccer, or pond hockey is your thing. Whatever it is, start slowly so you can build stamina and try to work out with people you are comfortable with. Whether you're kayaking, skiing, or going for long walks, you want to be proud of your achievement at the end of the day.

When beginning an exercise regimen, it is better to start out by setting your goals too low rather than too high. If you are exercising with other Peer Pressure Eaters, remember that you do not want to eat unhealthy foods after you are done working out. Instead, reward yourself for working out with something that is not food-oriented, such as giving yourself time to play a video game or watch a funny movie (while avoiding all the buttery popcorn!).

If you're a Peer Pressure Eater, you should:

- Eat at least one lunch and one dinner meal at home by yourself, sitting at the table.

- Drink a variety of low and no-calorie beverages (without artificial sweeteners) such as herbal tea, sparkling water, flavored water, or spa water.

- Look up restaurant menus online before you go out, pre-select what you are going to have, and stick to that choice.

Food for the Peer Pressure Eater

CLEAN PROTEINS:
organic chicken, turkey, beef, pork, wild fish, non-GMO soy proteins.

ALWAYS ORGANIC DIRTY DOZEN*:
apples, celery, strawberries, peaches, spinach, nectarines, grapes, sweet bell peppers (red, orange, and yellow), potatoes, blueberries, lettuce, kale.

*These fruits and vegetables contain the most pesticides when traditionally grown, so always choose organic.

Eating Strategies for the Peer Pressure Eater

Meal planning and social planning is key for the Peer Pressure Eater. Every Sunday, sit down with your calendar and look at your upcoming week to determine what events are on your schedule and which ones involve food. It could be a lunch meeting, happy hour, a kid's soccer game—anything where you typically eat or are triggered to eat should be included on your schedule/ meal plan. Once you have your events recorded, look at the open or "at home" days and write in a protein source for dinner to fill in the blanks. Be sure to include fish at least twice, but beef and pork for a total of no more than three times for both; you may want to include "Meatless Mondays" (or some variant of that) as a vegetarian day.

Next, jot down some recipe ideas or meals made with each protein—then go back and plan your lunches, which could be based on leftovers or sandwiches. Finally, write down breakfast items and make your grocery list for the week. You can shop once or pick up things a few times during the week, depending on your schedule. This will get easier and easier each week that you plan out your meals, and there are numerous programs and apps available that can assist you with meal planning if you need the help.

Now that you have an outline of what you will eat at home, look at your social functions and note what you are planning to eat at each one; as the week goes on, really try to stick to your food rules—organic, clean proteins and produce. You may decide that it's better to bring your own salad to the company luncheon and use whatever protein is provided to pair with it, or opt to bring half a sandwich or a high quality protein bar from home to your child's soccer game instead of being tempted by a preservative and fat-filled hot dog while you're there. The goal is to create and lead a new clean and healthy food trend among your peers rather than be a follower of poor food choices. You will notice that your peers will start paying attention to the fact that you are taking great care in how you nourish your body and they will be less likely to encourage you to eat junk. Furthermore, the more you stick to your food rules, the better you will feel and the more confidence you will have in social situations.

As you encounter each social situation during the week, really think about and savor each bite of food you are putting in your mouth. One of the problems with being a Peer Pressure eater is that you are talking and socializing so much that you're not *tasting* your food.

When you are at a lunch or dinner, don't take too much food at once and take a slow bite of each item to see if you like how it tastes. Give yourself permission to leave a food item on your plate that simply doesn't taste good to you.

It's a good idea for Peer Pressure Eaters to keep a food journal. This will help you see how closely you are able to stick to your meal plan, allow you to record your choices in social situations, and monitor your progress. Create a list of the people, places, and foods that trigger you the most, and consider this each Sunday when you are planning your meals. There may be some people you determine are better to invite over to your home, where you are in control of the food, than to go out with or to visit at their home. Ultimately, this process will put you in more control of your choices, and you won't feel like you've been pressured!

Download a FREE meal-planning template here:
http://www.PsychedtobeSkinny.com

Skinny Tips for the Peer Pressure Eater

Be a "two-fisted" drinker at parties—and one of the drinks needs to be water or sparkling water! Peer Pressure Eaters tend to drink too many cocktails. You can reduce the amount you drink by making sure to always be drinking a glass of water at the same time. (This also makes it more difficult to have your "free hand" grabbing chips or nuts or other foods.)

Begin researching and preparing healthy and clean eating recipes. This will help you find foods to prepare as well as transform your mindset to be the new clean-eating leader among your peers.

Recipe for the Peer Pressure Eater

Selecting organic foods may be slightly more expensive but when you taste how flavorful it is you will realize it is worth it. You will also find that you are satisfied with less food because you are choosing wholesome, fresh foods instead of processed foods.

Chicken with Tomatoes, Fennel & Capers

PREP TIME: 5 minutes
COOK TIME: 20 minutes
SERVINGS: 2

Ingredients

1 large boneless, skinless chicken breast, sliced in strips
1 teaspoon olive oil
1 fennel bulb, chopped (approximately one cup)
1 tablespoon chopped shallots
1 clove garlic, minced
3 Roma tomatoes, diced
8-10 leaves flat leaf parsley
1 teaspoon Italian seasoning
2 tablespoons capers, drained
Salt and pepper, to taste

Instructions

Spray a 12-inch nonstick skillet with cooking spray; heat over medium-high heat. Add chicken, garlic, and gingerroot and stir-fry 2 to 3 minutes, or until chicken is brown.

Add onion, carrots, 3/4 cup of the broth, the soy sauce, and the sugar. Cover and cook over medium heat 5 minutes, stirring twice.

Add broccoli, mushrooms, and bell pepper. Cover and

cook about 5 minutes more, stirring occasionally, until chicken is no longer pink in center and vegetables are crisp-tender.

Mix cornstarch with remaining 1/4 cup broth; stir into chicken mixture. Cook, stirring frequently, until sauce is thickened. Serve over steamed cabbage.

Nutritional Facts per serving:
Calories 180
Total Fat 3g
Saturated Fat 1g
Cholesterol 66mg
Sodium 397mg
Total Carbs 11g
Dietary Fiber 4g
Sugar 4g
Protein 28g

9

The I Deserve It Eater

The I Deserve It Eater eats as a celebration of what they have accomplished that day, that week, or that month ("I worked hard today, therefore I deserve food") as well as when things do not go well in their life ("I deserve to eat because I've had a rough day"). Often the I Deserve It Eater was given food as a young child as a reward when they won their baseball game or did well on a test, or as consolation when they lost or did poorly. The I Deserve It Eater will often come home from a particularly good day—or a particularly bad day—at work or school and start eating right away.

The I Deserve It Eater looks for other eaters who like to celebrate or commiserate over food—people they can eat with when something has gone either right or wrong in their lives.

They also like special events and holidays—birthday parties, Thanksgiving, Christmas, Hanukah, Kwanzaa—because they give them a reason to eat large amounts of (often unhealthy) food. The I Deserve It Eater does not always eat large quantities of food in front of other people; sometimes they may indulge in eating after everyone has left as a reward for having cooked a nice meal or hosted a great holiday or birthday dinner. This type of eater often feels that they are being watched or judged by others, so they often prefer to eat in solitude—then they feel guilty the next day and vow not to eat like that again. When the next disappointment or celebration comes along, however, the I Deserve It Eater overindulges again.

If you're an I Deserve It Eater, you need to:

- Figure out what emotions you are having when you eat.

- Learn to not stuff your emotions down in the form of food; instead, teach yourself to confront people and issues that are bothering you.

- Find other hobbies and things that you enjoy besides eating.

- Determine what time of the day you mainly eat, and plan non-food-related activities to engage in during that time.

- Refrain from taking food home with you when you go out to eat so you won't be tempted to eat it when you get home.

- Try calling a friend or relative that you are close to for support when you're feeling sad or depressed instead of turning to food.

- Look at food labels and opt for healthier choices.

- Talk to a therapist about your emotions.

- Keep active.

- Eat something healthy before you go to a celebration; you will be less tempted to eat foods that are unhealthy.

Cognitive Behavioral Exercises for the I Deserve It Eater

The I Deserve it Eater needs to be cognizant of what and when they think they are deserving of food. Writing down times and days when they need to replace their desire to eat with something positive will empower them. When you are at a party or have had a rough day at work, try to take comfort in staying away from the food table—and before you go to a party, have a healthy snack so you don't end up overindulging. When you do eat at a party, try to make smart choices; reach for the fruit and veggie trays before you reach for desserts or other fattening foods.

If you find yourself eating because you have had a bad day, you should head out to the gym or do some aerobic activity prior to eating. Exercising can often make you feel less hungry. People who work out also tend to feel less anger and frustration than people who do not work out, which can help with your bad eating habits.

Solution-Focused Exercises for the
I Deserve It Eater

If you could get any wish granted about your relationship with food, what would it look be? Would you like to be able to go to a party and have fun without stuffing yourself with unhealthy food? Would you like to make healthy choices and go home from every event you attend happy with your eating decisions? Would you like to figure out healthier ways to feel better when you've had a bad day? Do you wish you could find a healthy choice and stick to it when you go out to your favorite restaurant? Do you wish you could eat smaller portions when you are out celebrating?

You have the ability and strength of mind to do all of the above. Make a mental note of how guilty or frustrated you feel about yourself the day after you indulge in too much unhealthy food. Make feeling good about yourself and your appearance your ultimate goal. If you do this consistently, you will be able to maintain a healthy and happy lifestyle that others will want to emulate.

Physical Exercise for the
I Deserve it Eater

As always, check with your medical doctor to rule out any possible medical issues that might be causing you to eat overeat, such as hypothyroidism, before starting a new exercise regimen. Once your doctor has ruled out physical illness, make sure you let also let them know if you have been feeling overly emotional or stressed out lately. If you have, they may want to refer you to a therapist who can help you get in touch with why you are overeating or binge eating.

Going to the gym or working out after a frustrating day is the best option for the I Deserve It Eater—kickboxing, running, or fast biking are all good options. The I Deserve It Eater needs to know when to work out alone and when to work out with others. If you are frustrated because you didn't stand up to your boss after being yelled at or were bullied in school that day, you may want to work out so you don't take your stuffed-down emotions out on undeserving participants. If you're in a good mood, however, you may wish to participate in a group activity; a friendly game of football, hockey, or soccer maybe just what you need.

Keep in mind that these are exercise *suggestions*; you know yourself better than we do so do what works for you. It could be walking and talking with a trusted friend or relative, or it could be sledding with your family. Whatever it is, make sure it's something that you enjoy!

If you're an I Deserve It Eater, you should:

- Avoid buffets and other all-you-can-eat situations.

- Drink 1–2 cups of green tea daily (unsweetened).

- Eat yogurt with live cultures or take a pre/probiotic daily.

- Refrain from eating or drinking anything after 8:00 p.m. except a calorie-free beverage*.

*Do not drink anything with artificial sweeteners. Stevia is acceptable in moderation.

Food for the I Deserve It Eater

SUPER FOODS:
beans, blueberries, broccoli, oats, oranges, pumpkin, salmon, spinach, tomatoes, walnuts, flaxseeds, cruciferous vegetables (broccoli, cabbage, brussels sprouts), citrus fruits, soy, sweet potatoes.

SUPER DRINKS:
green tea, pomegranate juice*, acai berry juice*, electrolyte-enhanced water, coconut water*, aloe water*.

*Limit juices and calorie-containing beverages to two 8-ounce servings daily.

Meals for the I Deserve It Eater

The I Deserve It Eater tends to have an "all or nothing" mindset and can easily justify to themselves that they deserve to splurge and overindulge on multiple food items in one sitting. The I Deserve It Eater needs to change their mindset and think about the fact that what they deserve is to *nourish their body*, not to feed it decadent high-fat, high-sugar, and high-sodium foods in excess. This is why Super Foods and Super Drinks are excellent choices for the I Deserve It Eater—they're high-nutrient foods that your body needs and that you can feel good about eating.

You will also want to change what your idea of a splurge is. For you, a splurge at a restaurant likely consists of a high-fat appetizer (nachos, onion rings, a creamy cheesy dip for bread); a high-calorie/high-fat meal with soup, salad, and bread (Chicken Alfredo, beef enchiladas, fried chicken); a dessert; and two calorie-filled cocktails (daiquiris, mai tais, margaritas). As you can see, every one of these courses is an indulgent splurge! Look at other ways to splurge instead — maybe order wild game, fish, or a complex-flavored (yet healthful) dish that you wouldn't make for yourself at home. Or perhaps your splurge can be sharing dessert with the table; that way you get to enjoy a few bites without overindulging.

The I Deserve It Eater might want to create a dining experience with candles, music, fine china, and a menu of Super Foods — because you do deserve to pamper yourself! (You may want to review some of the tips for the Situational Eater, too.) Be cautious and careful with fringe foods: alcohol, appetizers, and dessert. It's easy to overdo it on fringe foods because they tend to be the first line of indulgence and therefore easily rationalized as being things that you "deserve." If there is a particular appetizer you want to enjoy, maybe order it as an entrée — and if there is a dessert on the menu that you know you can't resist, remember that you are not obligated to eat a four-course meal in order to have dessert and that it might be a better strategy to have a broth-based soup, small salad, and then the dessert! (Please don't do this often, however, or you won't get adequate nutrients.) Once your mind switches over to realizing that you deserve nourishing, wholesome, and fabulous-tasting food in proportions that meet your lifestyle and energy, you will begin to feel better about yourself overall and not feel the need to reward yourself with food

Skinny Tips for the I Deserve It Eater

Allow yourself a 100–200 calorie "treat" a few days per week. This is your chance to be slightly indulgent without going overboard; it will help you learn to click your brain away from eating it ALL. This way you aren't depriving yourself but you are learning moderation.

Access a FREE list of 100-calorie snacks here:
www.PsychedtobeSkinny.com

Recipe for the I Deserve It Eater

This version of Beurre Blanc sauce uses less butter than the traditional version, making it lower in fat and calories, and is a delicious addition to halibut. Prepare the sweet potato cubes first, then prepare the halibut while they are baking.

Grilled Halibut with Thyme Beurre Blanc and Sweet Potato Cubes

PREP TIME: 10 minutes
COOK TIME: 20 minutes
SERVINGS: 4

Ingredients

2/3 cup dry white wine
1/2 shallot, chopped
1/2 teaspoon whole black peppercorns
2 tablespoons fresh thyme leaves
3 tablespoons butter, cut into small pieces
1 teaspoon fresh thyme, chopped
4 6-oz. halibut fillets
1/4 teaspoon kosher salt
1/4 teaspoon freshly ground black pepper
1 teaspoon olive oil

Instructions

Beurre Blanc Sauce

Combine first four ingredients in a small, heavy saucepan over medium-high heat; bring to a boil. Cook until liquid is reduced to 2 tablespoons (about 9 minutes).

Remove from heat; strain through a fine sieve over a measuring cup, pressing mixture to release liquid. Discard solids. Return liquid to pan.

Add butter, one piece at a time, stirring with a whisk until butter is incorporated. Stir in thyme.

Halibut

Sprinkle halibut evenly with salt and ground pepper.

Heat a large grill pan over medium-high heat. Add olive oil.

Add fish to pan; cook 5 minutes on each side or until desired degree of doneness.

Place fish filets on plate and drizzle with sauce. Garnish with lemon wedge.

Nutrition Facts per serving:
Calories 242
Total Fat 10.7g
Saturated Fat 5.9g
Cholesterol 99mg
Sodium 303mg
Total Carbs 2.3g
Dietary Fiber 0.4g
Sugar 1g
Protein 29.1g

Roasted Sweet Potato Cubes

PREP TIME: 10 minutes
COOK TIME: 30 minutes
SERVINGS:

Ingredients

2 medium-sized sweet potatoes, peeled
1-2 tablespoons extra virgin olive oil
2 teaspoons paprika (more if desired)
Salt and pepper, to taste

Instructions

Preheat oven to 400 degrees.

Dice the potatoes into 1-inch cubes. Place the cubes in a medium-sized bowl, drizzle with olive oil, and season with paprika, salt, and pepper. Toss with hands to coat evenly and arrange in a single layer on a baking sheet.

Roast for about 30 minutes, or until tender, but slightly crispy in the outside. Stir once or twice during roasting.

Remove from oven and serve.

Nutrition Facts per serving:
Calories 97
Total Fat 4.5g
Saturated Fat 0.6g
Cholesterol 0mg
Sodium 424.2mg
Total Carbs 13.4g
Dietary Fiber 2g
Sugar 2.8g
Protein 1g

10

The Big-Boned Eater

The Big-Boned Eater eats because it has been engrained in them since they were young that they are built big-boned and therefore have no control over their weight. Often the Big-Boned Eater comes from a family whose members are large in stature and who treat food as a form of love or as an extension of their affection for one another. They may feel peer pressure from the rest of their family to eat large amounts of food, causing them to be overweight—though they may see it as a genetic problem ("My mom, dad, and siblings are all big people, therefore I am destined to be a big person as well.")

Often the Big-Boned Eater will order large amounts of food at a restaurant and explain to those around them that they have to order a lot of food because they are "big-boned." The Big-Boned Eater will often hear things like, "Eat, eat, you are getting too skinny," or "Is that all you're going to eat? I made this especially for you because I know it's your favorite!" from their relatives—something that makes them feel as if they will hurt someone's feelings if they do not eat large masses of food. The Big-Boned Eater often feels large amounts of guilt for not eating; they will frequently eat even when they're full to please others. Even when they're alone, they'll often eat large portions out of habit.

If the Big-Boned Eater loses weight, they often fall under the scrutiny of other Big-Boned Eaters ("What, you're too good to eat my food?"). A spouse or a significant other will sometimes even prompt a Big-Boned Eater to eat more because they don't want them to lose weight, either because they crave homeostasis because they are also a Big-Boned Eater and would like their partner to eat and enjoy food with them, or because of insecurity—they're scared that if their partner loses weight they will leave them.

If you're a Big-Boned Eater, you need to:

- Let other Big-Boned Eaters know that you plan to eat less and eat a better diet so you can become a healthier person.

- Not feel guilty when others are trying to get you to eat more.

- Put your health needs first.

- Talk to a therapist if you continue feeling guilty for not overeating.

- Know that you can be an inspiration to other Big-Boned Eaters.

- Not succumb to the peer pressure that may come from other Big-Boned Eaters trying to get you to maintain your "big-boned" mentality.

- See how healthy, fit people inspire themselves.

- Stop telling yourself that you're a Big-Boned Eater.

- Try not to bring the "big-boned" mentality into the next generation. If you have or are planning to have children, break the cycle now. Heart disease is the number one killer in the United States.

- Plan a healthy exercise regime when you become active; you will want to lose weight once you start exercising.

Cognitive Behavioral Exercises for the Big-Boned Eater

The Big-Boned Eater needs to journal the times they overeat and what they ate when they did and they need to try to cut their portions down small amounts at a time. Try eating three-fourths of what you usually eat for meals for two weeks. After two weeks, see if you can eat half of what you usually do at mealtimes. Use a smaller plate to trick your stomach into thinking that it is getting just as much food as before. Explain to friends, family, and/or your significant other that you will be eating smaller portions and healthier meals, and ask each Big-Boned Eater in your life — individually — if they will support you in your endeavor to become a healthier you. If you have feelings of guilt over your eating habits, write down how you feel and where the guilt is stemming from. Process this by yourself, with a trusted loved one, or with a professional.

Solution-Focused Exercises for the Big-Boned Eater

In a perfect world, what would your weight and shape be? How would you like others to look at and perceive you? If you were not a Big-Boned Eater, what would your life be like? Would you have more energy to do things like bike with your friends or play with your kids? Would you spend less time eating and more time taking walks or going for a jog? Would you be able to rock the outfits your non-"big-boned" friends can wear? Would you no longer hear "Oh, you have such a pretty face"? You deserve to show the whole world—including yourself—that you're not a "big-boned" person. Once you get to your ideal, healthy weight, you will be the fabulous you on the inside and on the outside.

Physical Exercise for the Big-Boned Eater

Before starting a new exercise regimen check with your medical doctor as you will want to make sure you are heart healthy. Have your cholesterol checked; if you have high cholesterol, you will be advised about what not to eat and may be advised to take medication as well. You should also rule out diabetes and hypertension before starting a new exercise plan.

You may want to start out slow when you begin exercising—going on a short walk around the block to begin with, then building up to running or biking. Big-Boned Eaters sometimes feel self-conscious at the gym; you may want use an exercise video instead, so you can exercise in the comfort of your own home. Make sure that you do not reward yourself with an unhealthy snack after exercising.

If you are social and want to join a biking club or a volleyball or basketball team, try joining a beginner's group to get in shape before jumping into a more advanced level. You don't want to become discouraged early on by people that you may not be able to keep up with. As you start to eat less and exercise more, your self-confidence will build. At that point, try working out in a gym and seeing what types of things interest you. Most gyms and fitness studios will let you work out free for the first week; use this to see if you would like to invest in a gym membership or if you would rather invest in some exercise equipment for your home. Remember to bring your tunes and a headset so you can listen to music or watch your favorite television show while you exercise.

If you are a younger Big-Boned Eater, try establishing friendships with active kids in your neighborhood. Playing neighborhood games is one of the best ways to have fun and burn off calories at the same time. Try biking or walking your dog, if you have one. Keep busy around the house—your parents will love the help. See if any elderly neighbors need their walks shoveled or their grass mowed—you will get exercise and feel good all around because you've done a good deed for someone.

Exercise can be more fun if it's a family affair. As an example, I started horseback riding lessons with my ten-year-old daughter and we both love it. And don't forget to change up your exercise routine so you don't get bored. Try biking one day, rollerblading the next (remember your helmet and pads), and running the day after that. Adults may want to try Pilates, Zumba, or hot yoga to tone their muscles. If you look around at your options, I guarantee you will find some activities you enjoy. If you can, try to get some other Big-Boned Eaters to join you—but don't let yourself become discouraged or disheartened if they are not ready to make the commitment that you have made. Enjoy the healthy, not-so-big-boned person you turn into as you grow more active. You will be an inspiration to many!

Download our FREE "Yoga Basics" PDF here:
www.PsychedtobeSkinny.com

If you're a Big-Boned Eater, you should:

- Start every meal with a broth-based vegetable soup (no starches), a large green salad, or a plate of raw vegetables.

- Limit your snacking (wait at least three hours after eating before having a snack).

- Reduce the number of fast food meals you eat each week, with the ultimate goal of eliminating fast food from your diet altogether.

Food for the Big-Boned Eater

LOW-CALORIE "FILLER FOOD" LEAFY GREENS: lettuces (romaine, butter/Bibb, endive, escarole, iceberg, red or green leaf, frisee, radicchio, mesclun), other leafy greens (spinach, arugula, cabbage, chard, collard, mustard, beet, dandelion, kale, watercress).

HIGH WATER CONTENT VEGETABLES: broccoli, carrots, cauliflower, celery, cucumber, eggplant, bell peppers, radish, zucchini, tomato.

HIGH WATER CONTENT FRUITS*:
watermelon, cantaloupe, honeydew melon, grapefruit, oranges, peaches, pineapple, strawberries, raspberries.

*Limit to three 1/2-cup servings per day.

Meals for the Big-Boned Eater

The primary goal for the Big-Boned Eater is to start shrinking your stomach and at the same time consciously tell yourself that you are satisfied with the amount of food you are eating. Because you have likely been overfeeding yourself with very calorically dense foods for years, you are going to need to reprogram how you physically respond to food and allow your stomach to feel slightly *empty* after meals.

A great way to illustrate how Big-Boned Eaters can approach this is to use real food examples. A typical Big-Boned Eater meal could be a super burrito, chips and salsa, and a 24-oz. soda or other sugary drink—a whopping 2,400 calories in total! Compare that to the 675 calories found in a meal consisting of a mixed green salad with avocado and light dressing, chicken breast, brown rice, green beans, strawberries, and a chocolate square. High-calorie foods (such as burritos), unlike nutrient and fiber-rich foods (such as salad, chicken, and brown rice), don't take up as much space in your stomach, which can result in overeating. If you're used to eating this way, like the Anxious Eater, your ability to distinguish between satisfied, full, and stuffed is probably impaired.

Satisfied ➜ Full ➜ Stuffed

You may need to rely on food facts (i.e., how many calories in a meal) more than a feeling of fullness for several weeks as you learn to eat less calorically dense foods. "Filler foods"—foods that are low in calories but high in nutrients—will be a big help during this process because they'll help take up some of the volume of your stomach so you can have a feeling of "fullness" without overindulging. This can be an effective tool when dining with family members that still have the Big Boned Eater mentality: fill your plate up with a huge salad and protein, and eat slowly. You will likely discover your family members will eat two helpings in the same time that you eat one. Remember, if you finish before they do, they are more likely to encourage you to "get more," so concentrate on slowing down.

You will want to avoid high-fat proteins and other high-fat foods. These foods aren't nutrient-dense enough to fill up your stomach but they will add a significant amount of calories to your daily count. Examples of high-fat foods to avoid include: bacon, sausage, hot dogs, cheese, deep-fried foods, donuts and pastries, regular and premium ice cream, heavy cream gravies and sauces, potato and tortilla chips, mayonnaise, and most salad dressings.

Skinny Tips for the Big-Boned Eater

Replace one meal per day with a high-quality meal replacement shake—one with fiber in it—at least four days per week. This will help you nourish your body with the nutrients it needs while still allowing your stomach to shrink.

Recipe for the Big-Boned Eater

This salad is perfect for the Big-Boned Eater because the potatoes give it a little bit of carbohydrates, but it's still loaded with veggies and lean protein. (Feel free to substitute salmon or shrimp for the tuna, if you prefer.) Make a large batch of the dressing and keep it on hand for other salads!

Green Salad with Seared Tuna & Lemon-Caper Dressing

PREP TIME: 20 minutes
COOK TIME: 10 minutes
SERVINGS: 4

Ingredients

For Salad

3/4 cup French green beans, trimmed, cut into 1-inch pieces
1 tablespoon extra-virgin olive oil, divided
1 cooked Yukon Gold potato, diced
1 large head Bibb lettuce, leaves torn
1/2 cup fresh basil leaves
1 cup grape tomatoes, halved lengthwise
1/2 cup red onion, thinly sliced
1/4 cup pitted Kalamata olives, halved lengthwise
2 hardboiled eggs, peeled and quartered
2 8-oz. tuna steaks
1/8 teaspoon sea salt
1/8 teaspoon black pepper, freshly ground

For Dressing

Juice of 2 lemons
1 tablespoon water
2 tablespoons extra virgin olive oil or grapeseed oil
1 tablespoon white wine vinegar
1/2 teaspoon sugar

1/8 teaspoon salt
1/8 teaspoon black pepper, freshly ground
1 garlic clove, minced
1 tablespoon capers

Instructions

For Salad

Cook green beans in boiling water 2 minutes or until crisp-tender. Drain and place in ice-water bath to cool. Drain thoroughly and set aside.

Heat a large nonstick skillet or cast iron skillet over medium-high heat. Add olive oil to pan; swirl to coat.

Sprinkle tuna with salt and pepper. Place tuna in the center of pan; place potatoes around the edges. Cook tuna 2 minutes on each side or until desired degree of doneness. Stir potatoes and cook until warm.

Remove tuna from pan and cut thin slices, across the grain. Arrange tuna on 4 plates.

Arrange lettuce and basil evenly on plates. Divide tomatoes, onion, olives, eggs, green beans, and potatoes among plates; top with tuna slices.

For Dressing

Combine lemon juice, water, vinegar, sugar, salt, pepper, and garlic in a small bowl.

Gradually add oil to the bowl, stirring constantly with a whisk. Stir in capers.
Drizzle evenly over salads.

Nutrition Facts per serving:
Calories 407
Total Fat 19g
Saturated Fat 3g
Cholesterol 137mg
Sodium 566mg
Total Carbs 18g
Dietary Fiber 4g
Sugar 5g
Protein 35g

Conclusion

Ninety percent of life is just showing up.
—Woody Allen

"I,_____, commit myself to a healthy lifestyle and will try to the best to my ability to succeed in upholding this commitment."

As someone who has made the decision to pursue a new, more healthy way of life, you must use the above statement as your mantra every day. Remember, there is no fast and easy way to lose weight—nor is there a fast and easy way to keep it off. This book isn't about a quick fix; it's about making a lifelong promise to yourself to change your food mood using Denise's cognitive tools and Susie's eating tips. It's about staying positive, getting that workout in, trying that healthy recipe, and making real lifestyle changes.

You may have to go the extra mile. You may have a love-hate relationship with the food choices and work-out plans this commitment will require you to make. But the key is to *just show up*. Make that healthy choice at the restaurant. Go on that walk or run. The more often you do these things, the easier it will become—and once you start seeing results, you'll be glad you've pushed through the hard part.

There are always a million excuses to avoid personal reflection time, not work out, or eat the foods that you know you will feel bad about eating later. Don't let yourself make those excuses. Instead, let yourself succeed at this venture. Once you do, your pride and sense of accomplishment will be astronomical, and all your efforts will be rewarded.

So get going. Make the commitment. *Show up*. We know you can do it.

Bonus Meal Plans

On the following pages you'll find sample meal plan ideas—for breakfast, lunch, and dinner—for each of the eating types we've discussed in this book. You'll notice that some of the meal items include a list of ingredients that can be used to easily put something together—a kind of "mini-recipe." Give them a try! All portion sizes mentioned are standardized. If any of the fruits we suggest below aren't currently available, feel free to substitute seasonal fruits.

Sample Meal Plan: The Depressed Eater

Breakfast

1 cup natural or steel-cut oatmeal, cooked
1 teaspoon flaxseed (whole or crushed)
1/2 cup blueberries
1 hardboiled egg

Lunch

Green apple
Ground turkey tacos:
- 2 corn tortillas
- 4 oz. ground turkey
- 2 tablespoons black beans
- lettuce
- tomato
- 1/2 avocado, split
- salsa

Dinner

Low-Carb Chicken, Broccoli & Mushroom Stir-Fry (see end
of Chapter 1 for recipe)
1 cup shredded cabbage
1 cup sliced strawberries

Sample Meal Plan: The Anxious Eater

Breakfast

Protein bar (12-20 grams protein)
1/3 cup cantaloupe cubes

Lunch

1 serving whole-grain crackers
1 orange
Chopped salad:
- 2 cups Romaine lettuce
- 3/4 cup diced turkey
- 1/3 bell pepper (any color)
- 1/4 cup shredded carrots
- 1/2 cup broccoli
- 1 tablespoon slivered almonds
- 2 tablespoons vinaigrette dressing

Dinner

Savory Bean & Spinach Soup (see end of Chapter 2 for recipe)
1 slice high-fiber bread
1 medium pear

Sample Meal Plan: The Situational Eater

Breakfast

6–8 oz. plain Greek yogurt
1/4 cup granola
1/2 cup mixed berries

Lunch

Greek Chicken Salad Pita Sandwich & Butternut Squash Soup (see end of Chapter 3 for recipe)
1 small apple

Dinner

4 oz. broiled trout with fresh lemon juice
1/2 cup quinoa
1 cup broccoli (raw or steamed)

Sample Meal Plan: The Bored Eater

Breakfast

Veggie egg scramble:
- 2 eggs
- zucchini
- mushroom
- tomato
- 1/3 avocado

1 slice dark rye toast
1 clementine

Lunch

1 serving whole-wheat pretzels
Spinach salad:
- 2 cups spinach
- 3 oz. cooked chicken breast (fresh or canned)
- 1/2 cup sliced strawberries
- 1/2 cup cherry tomatoes
- 1/2 cup diced cucumber
- 2 tablespoons light basil-balsamic dressing

Dinner

Salmon with Aromatic Spice Rub (see end of Chapter 4 for recipe)
1/2 cup brown rice or quinoa
5 large stalks asparagus, steamed

Sample Meal Plan: The Recently Dumped Eater

Breakfast

Protein smoothie:
- 1 scoop protein powder of any kind
- 1 cup almond milk
- 1/2 banana
- 1/2 cup strawberries
- 1 teaspoon peanut butter
- ice, if desired

Lunch

1 cup green salad with light dressing
15 grapes
Grilled chicken breast sandwich:
- 3 oz. grilled chicken breast
- whole-wheat bun or 2 slices whole-wheat bread
- 2 teaspoons olive oil mayonnaise
- 2 teaspoons Dijon mustard
- lettuce
- tomato

Dinner

Veggie plate appetizer:
- carrot sticks
- celery sticks
- radish
- cucumber
- balsamic vinegar (for dipping)

Slow Cooker Vegetable Casserole (see end of Chapter 5 for recipe)
1 small orange

Sample Meal Plan: The Fat is My Shelter Eater

Breakfast

3/4 cup low-fat cottage cheese
1 medium-size fresh peach, cubed
1 slice high-fiber seeded bread

Lunch

Zucchini Lime Turkey Burger (see end of Chapter 6 for recipe)
1/8 avocado, sliced
1/2 cup organic black beans
1 cup green salad with oil & vinegar dressing
1/2 cup honeydew melon, cubed

Dinner

4 oz. chicken breast (baked, grilled, or sautéed)
1/2 cup brown basmati rice
1 cup steamed green beans
6 dried apricot halves

Sample Meal Plan: The Period Eater

Breakfast

Vegan protein drink:
- 1–2 scoops vegan protein powder
- 1 cup coconut milk
- 1/2 teaspoon cinnamon
- ice, if desired

Lunch

Low-sodium vegetable soup
1 serving gluten-free crackers
1 small apple
1 cup tuna salad:
- 1 can White Albacore tuna
- 2 teaspoons olive oil
- 1/3 cup celery, diced
- fresh ground pepper

Dinner

Small green salad with lettuce and tomato, oil & vinegar dressing
Open-Faced Chicken & Pepper Sandwich (see end of Chapter 7 for recipe)
1 plum

Sample Meal Plan: The Peer Pressure Eater

Breakfast

Veggie omelet:
- 1 egg
- 2 egg whites
- spinach
- mushrooms
- tomato
- 1 oz. goat cheese

1 slice sprouted wheat bread
1 teaspoon local honey

Lunch

Mixed green salad with salmon:
- 2 cups mixed greens
- 3 oz. cooked fresh salmon (not farm-raised)
- 1/2 cup chopped asparagus, blanched
- 1/2 cup cherry tomatoes
- 1/8 avocado
- 1 teaspoon pine nuts
- 2 tablespoons garlic vinaigrette dressing

1/2 cup steamed lentils (hot or cold)
1 medium nectarine

Dinner

Chicken with Tomatoes, Fennel & Capers (see end of Chapter 8 for recipe)
1/2 cup brown rice or quinoa pasta
1 cup steamed broccoli

Remember, it's important for Peer Pressure Eaters to stick to organic, clean proteins and produce whenever possible.

Sample Meal Plan: The I Deserve It Eater

Breakfast

2 slices flaxseed bread (50–60 calories per slice)
2 teaspoons almond butter (one per slice)
1 poached egg

Lunch

1 veggie burger patty (no bun)
1 cup cabbage slaw:
- shredded cabbage
- shredded carrots
- diced red pepper
- 1 tablespoon rice wine vinegar
- 1 tablespoon olive oil
- fresh ground pepper
15 red grapes

Dinner

Grilled Halibut with Thyme Beurre Blanc and Sweet Potato Cubes (see end of Chapter 9 for recipe)
3/4 cup sautéed green beans

Sample Meal Plan: The Big-Boned Eater

Breakfast

1 1/2 cups low-calorie (less than 100 calories per cup)
breakfast cereal
3/4 cup skim milk
1/2 cup sliced strawberries
1 hardboiled egg

Lunch

Green Salad with Seared Tuna & Lemon-Caper Dressing (see
end of Chapter 10 for recipe)
1/2 cup sliced honeydew melon

Dinner

Large green salad:
- mixed greens
- tomato
- cucumber
- bell pepper
- mushrooms
4 oz. grilled chicken breast
1/2 cup wild and brown rice pilaf
1 cup steamed broccoli, cauliflower, and carrot

FREE bonuses
for readers of
Psyched to be Skinny

Receive the valuable bonuses that we describe in each chapter by visiting www.psychedtobeskinny.com. You will also learn about additional resources including our upcoming webinars, seminars, and workshops. If you enjoyed reading Psyched to be Skinny, we would love to hear from you!

Acknowledgments

Dr. Denise Wood

This book is dedicated to my son, Nick, daughter, Page, and husband, Jim—you are my heart, my love, my fun. Also for my mother, Connie, father, Dennis, and sister, Mandee Page, who never gave up on me—and finally, for my brother, Scott, who gave up on himself all too early. I love all of you more than the sky is high and the sea is deep.

Susie Garcia

Thank you to my Uncle Paul and Aunt Eileen who invited me to California, opened their home to me and helped me "start over" in 2006. You're the reason I was able to start down an amazing new path and meet my husband, Dave, who provides rock solid support for me and makes me laugh daily. A special thank you as well to my sisters, Deb and Kathy, and my mom and dad for helping and encouraging me in everything I do.

About the Authors

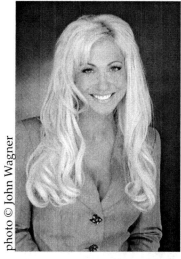

Dr. Denise Wood, MA, PsyD

Dr. Denise Wood is a doctor of clinical psychology with a master's degree from St. Mary's University in Minneapolis and a PsyD degree from the Illinois School of Professional Psychology, a school fully accredited by the American Psychological Association.

Dr. Wood is the founder of Wood Counseling Services, LLC where she performs relationship counseling for families and individuals alike. Prior to founding Wood Counseling Services, she held a Psychologist II position at the Minnesota Department of Corrections for many years. While there, she also served as a psychological profiler for the Moose Lake Rush Hostage Negotiations Team.

She also has experience with life coaching and executive coaching.

Dr. Wood lost her brother to suicide—due to mental illness—when he was forty years old, which inspired her to devote herself to promoting mental health wellness. Her goal is to ease the pain and suffering of others by using her medical expertise to offer great mental and physical health tips.

Dr. Wood is married to Dr. James Wood, MD, a gastroenterologist. She has two children and a furry friend named Sir Barkley. Visit her at www.drdenisewood.com.

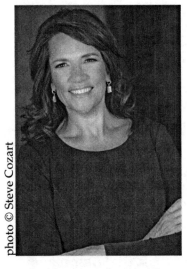

photo © Steve Cozart

Susie Garcia, RDN

Registered Dietitian Nutritionist Susie Garcia operates her private nutrition practice, Nutrition for Your Lifestyle, in the San Francisco Bay Area. Susie is an expert in weight management and works with her clients to change how they think about food at her practice, where she offers individual and family consultations and nutrition programs for businesses and organizations.

Susie completed her dietetic internship at Texas A&M University and received her bachelor's degree in nutrition from North Dakota State University, where she also minored in business administration and music. Early in her career, she received national recognition as a recipient of the Registered Young Dietitian of the Year Award from the Academy of Nutrition and Dietetics and Texas Dietetic Association. Before opening Nutrition for Your Lifestyle, she was an adjunct instructor at The Culinary Institute of America at Greystone in St. Helena, California, where she taught nutrition and food safety courses, and served as a media representative for the Texas and California Dietetic Associations, promoting food and nutrition messages via press releases, radio, and television appearances. Recently, she filmed two multi-video, nutrition-themed series for eHow.com.

Susie enjoys running, cooking, and playing her French Horn in a local community band. She lives in the Bay Area with her husband, Dave Garcia. Visit her at www.thesusiegarcia.com

Denise and Susie: The Story Behind the Book

If you're wondering how a Minnesota psychologist and a California dietitian got together to write a book: Denise and Susie attended Red River High School together in Grand Forks, North Dakota, and when they reconnected a few years ago at a mini-class reunion, they came up with the idea of writing a book together. When the timing was right, they rolled up their sleeves and got to work. *Psyched to Be Skinny* is the first of what they hope will be many more collaborations to come. Learn more at www.psychedtobeskinny.com!